Dedication

Thank you to Alexandria, Shane, and Emily.
You inspired us to start this journey and continue to fill our lives with joy and fulfillment!

Thank you to Dr. Dale Dangleben.
You inspire us to be creative and to take risks. Your energy and commitment to medicine is boundless and makes us strive to reach higher.

Thank you to our patients.
You inspire us to always be the best nurses we can be in giving care and helping to save lives.

Thank you to the children.
You inspire us to want to pass on the knowledge we have gained as nurses. Our hope is that our books will make you a little more comfortable as you enter the healthcare setting. We also hope you consider a career in healthcare where you have the ability to make a difference in lives every day. You are our future!

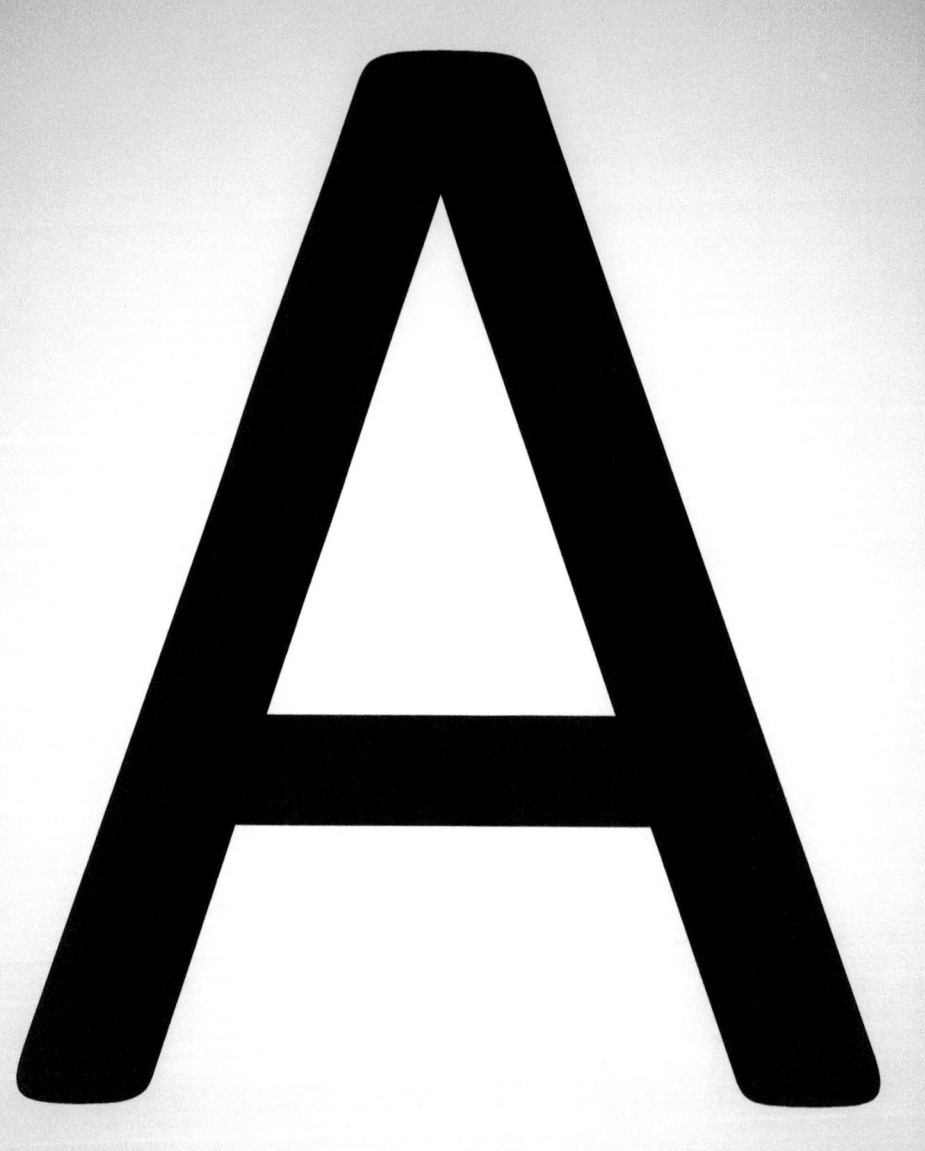

A: Ambulance

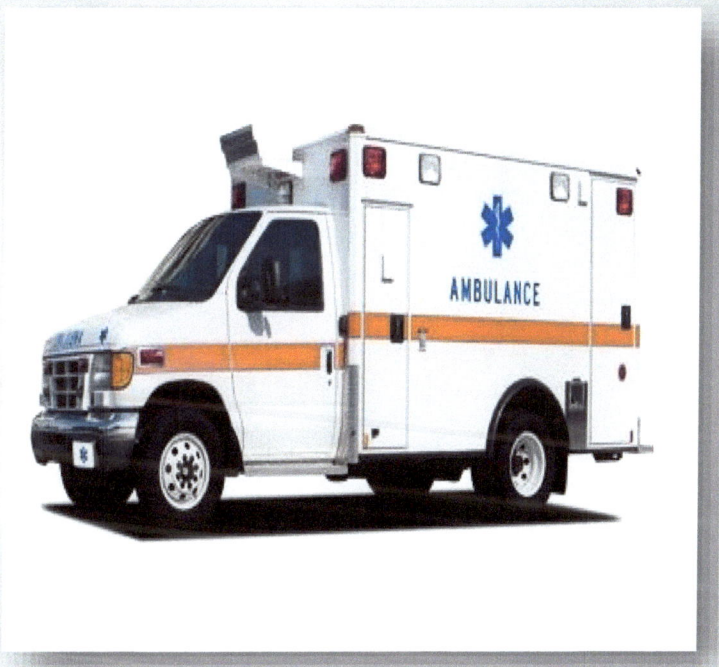

When you are sick or injured
Or are hurt from a bad fall

An ambulance will take you to the hospital
When it is 911 you call.

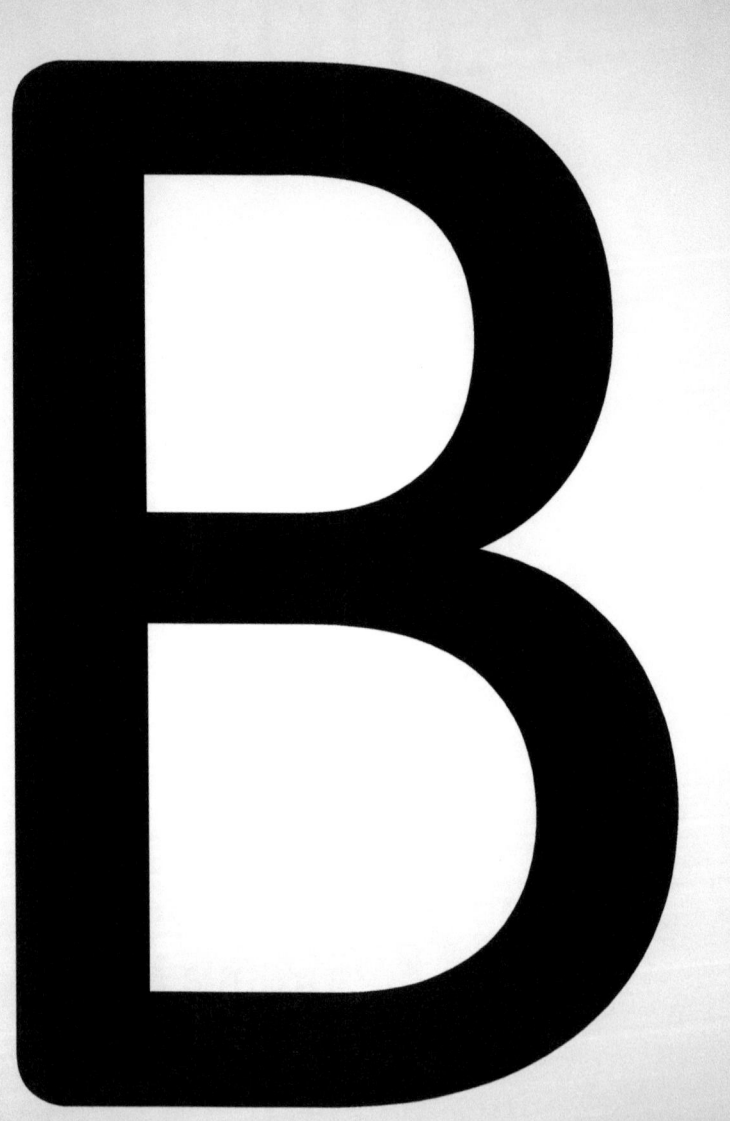

B: Bandage

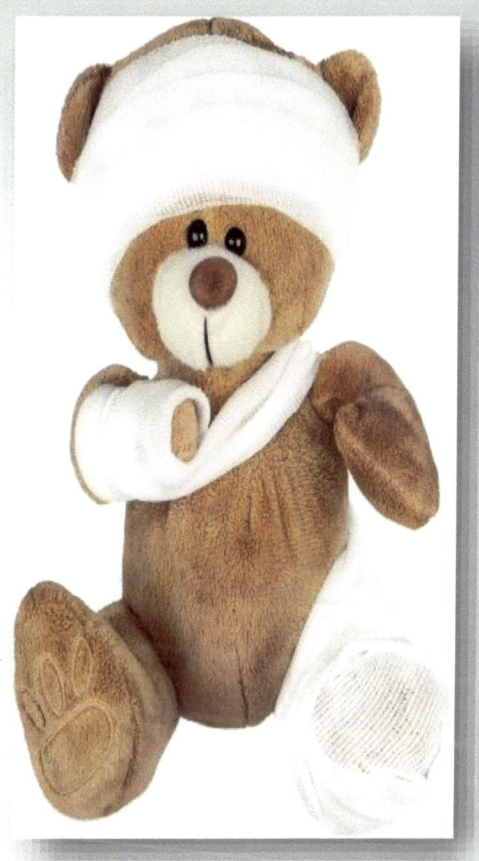

You can apply a bandage
When you get a cut or bite

Leave it on for a few days
And soon it will feel alright.

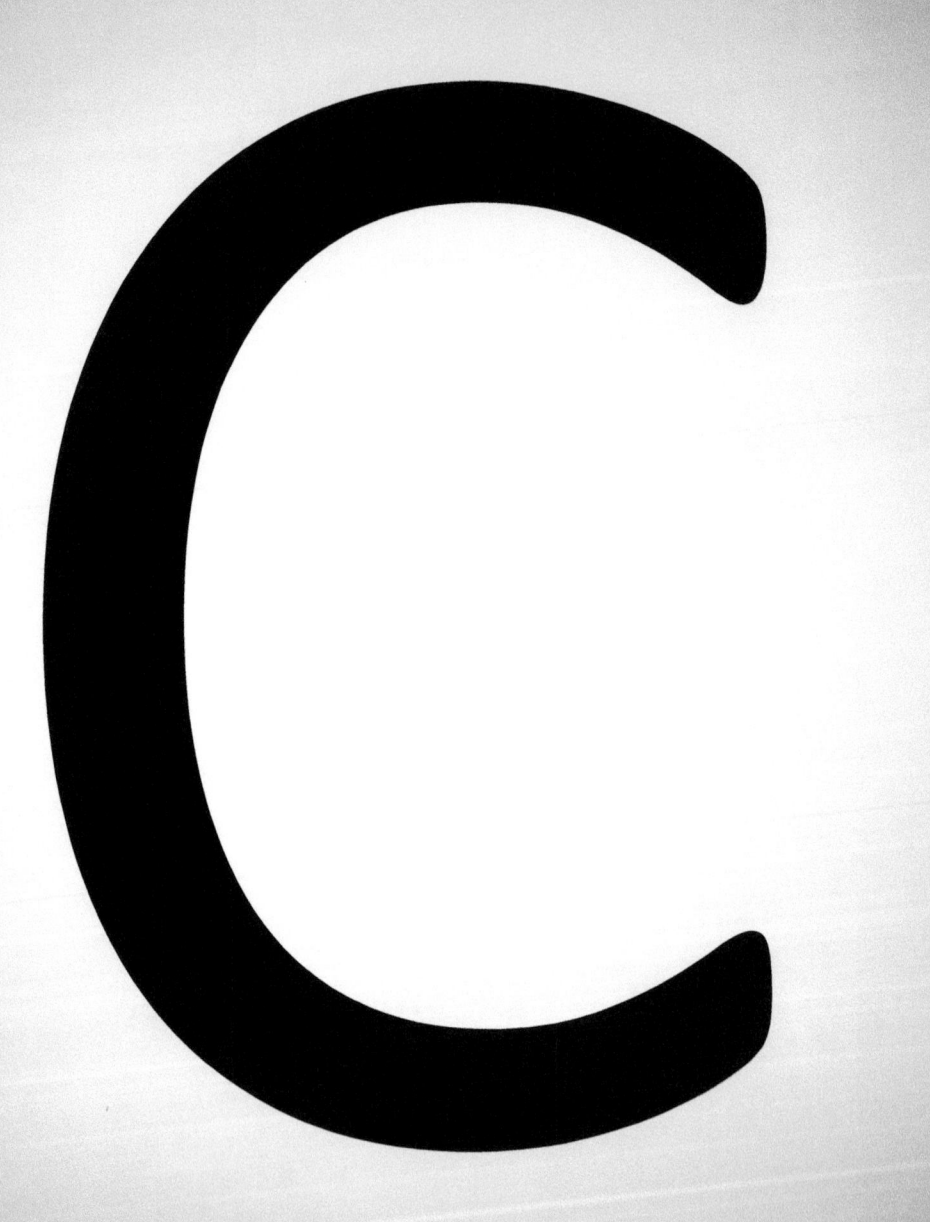

C: Cast

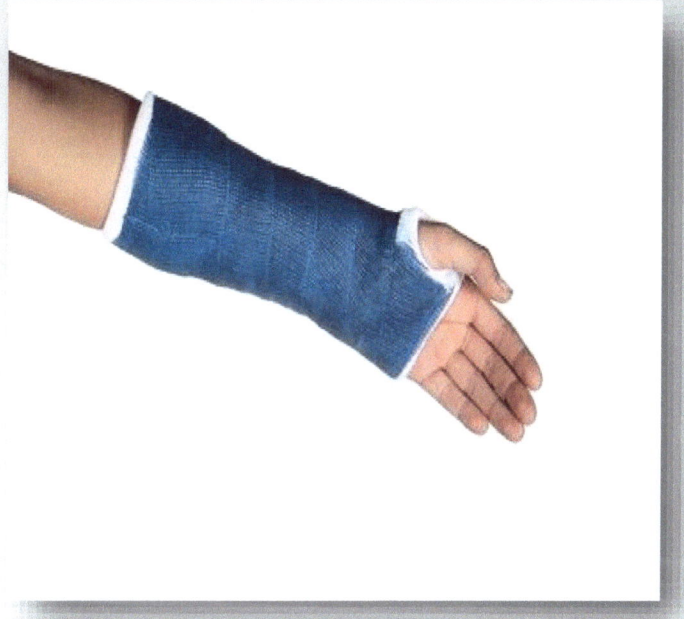

If you have a broken bone
You may need a cast

Get it signed by all your friends
It will heal real fast!

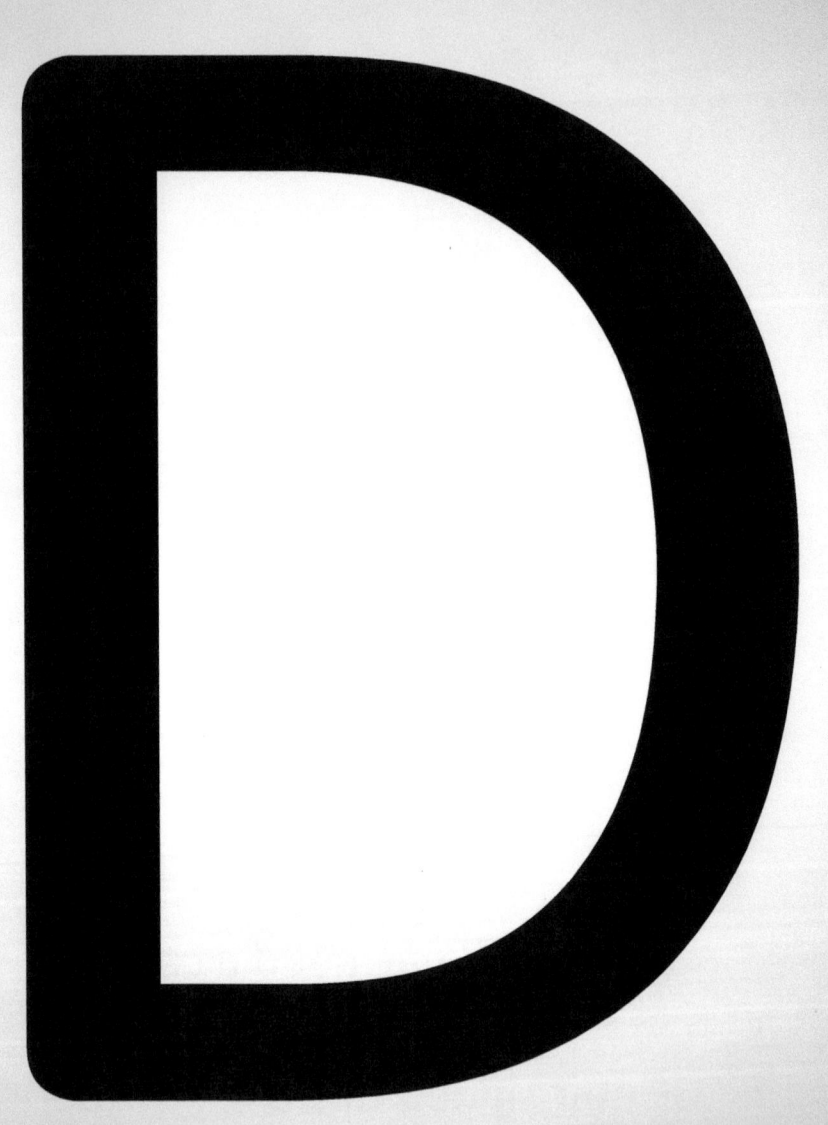

D: Doctor

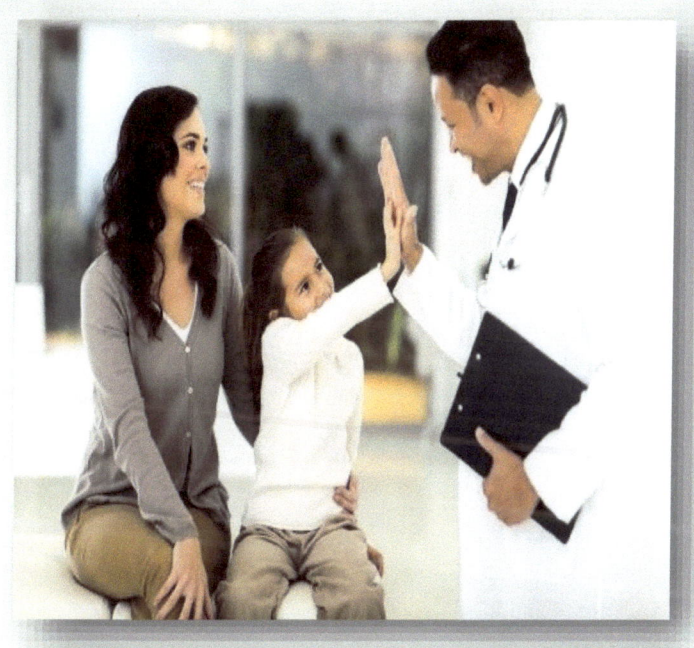

A doctor examines you at your appointment if you are well or sick
Developing a treatment plan that will be an excellent fit

Your relationship will keep growing strong
Because they will help you when something is wrong.

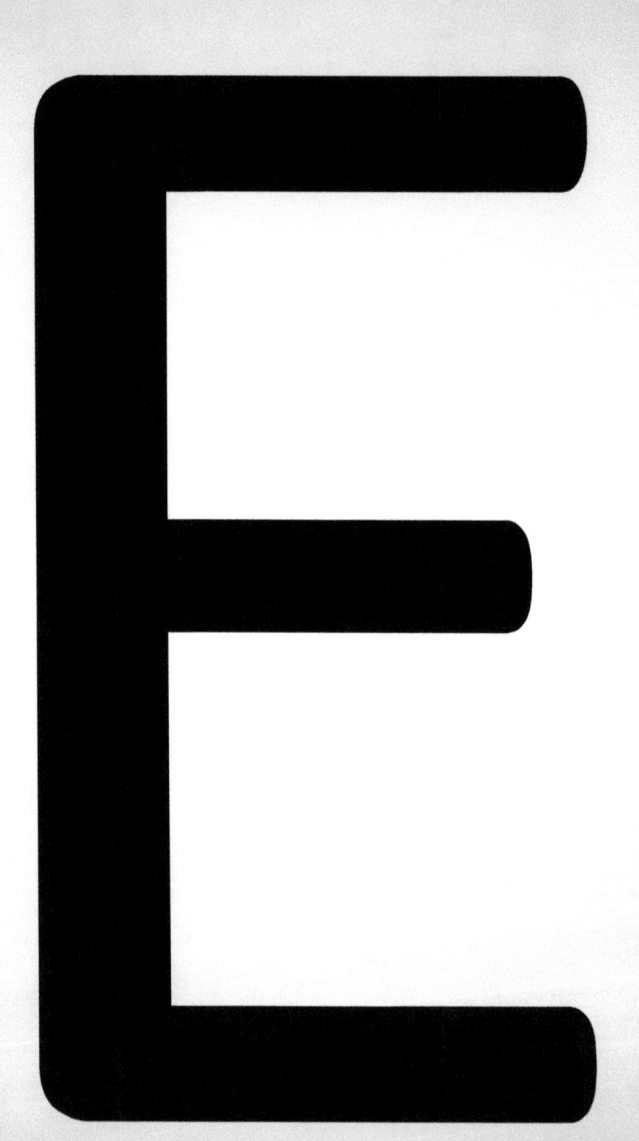

E: Eye drop

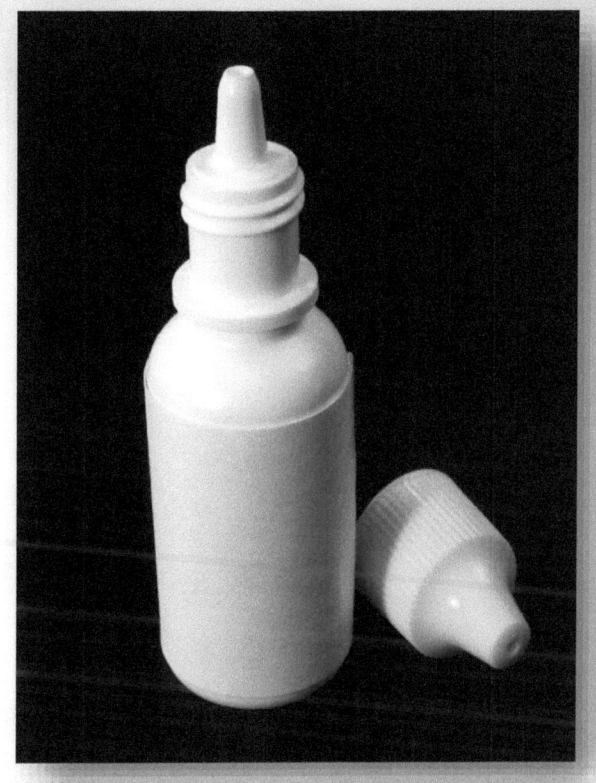

If your eyes are painful
Are swollen or are red

Your doctor will prescribe some eye drops
And send you home to bed.

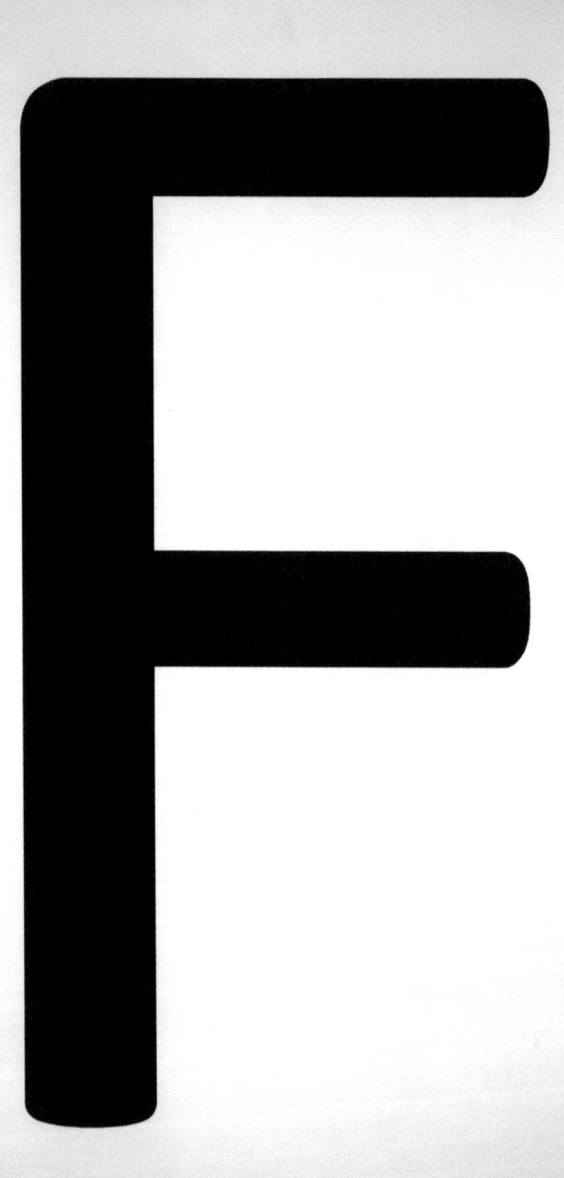

F: Fracture

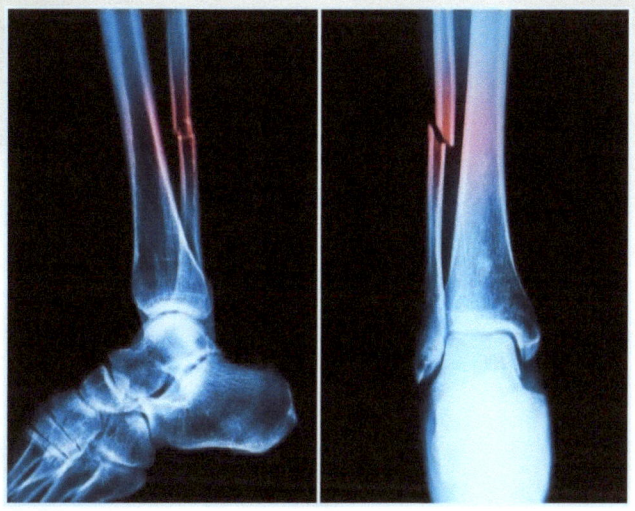

A fracture is a break in your bone
From your leg to your arm to your finger alone

The treatment maybe surgery or applying a cast
This is all done for healing that will last.

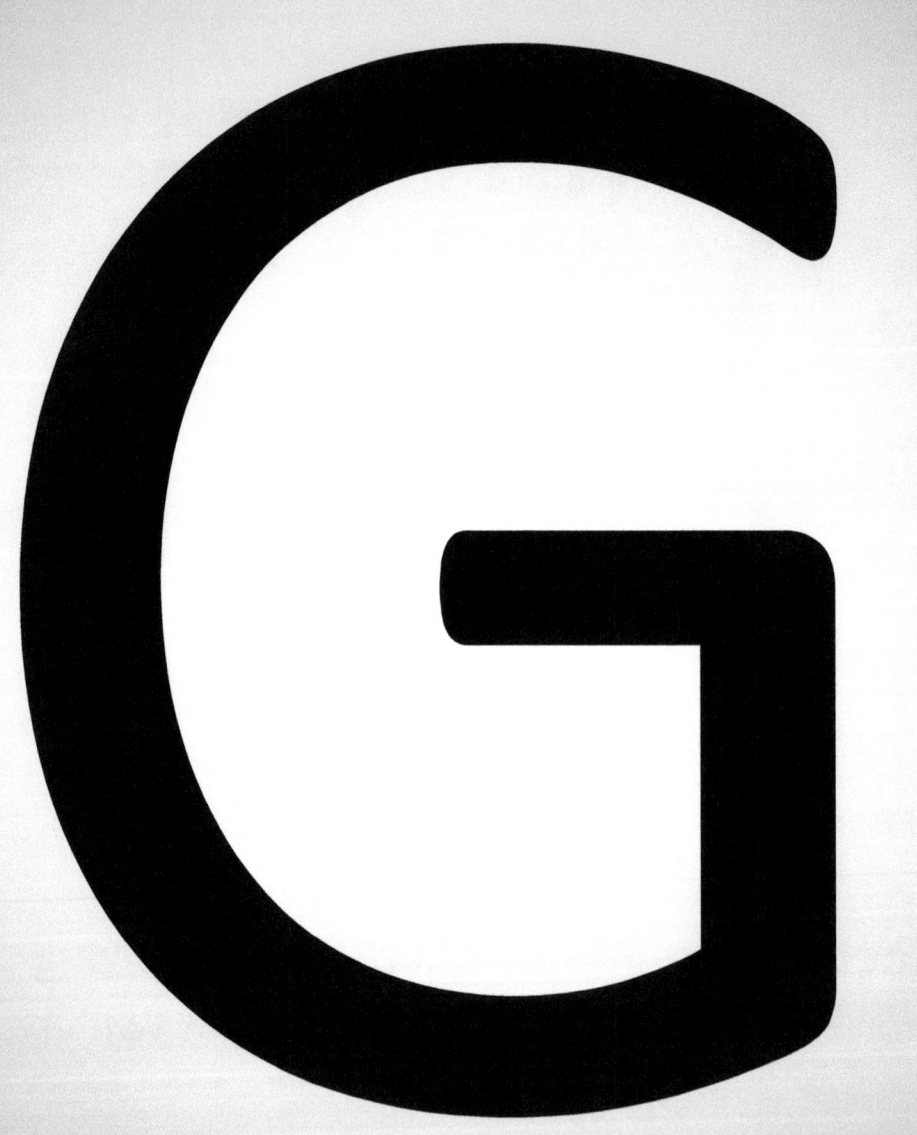

G: Gloves

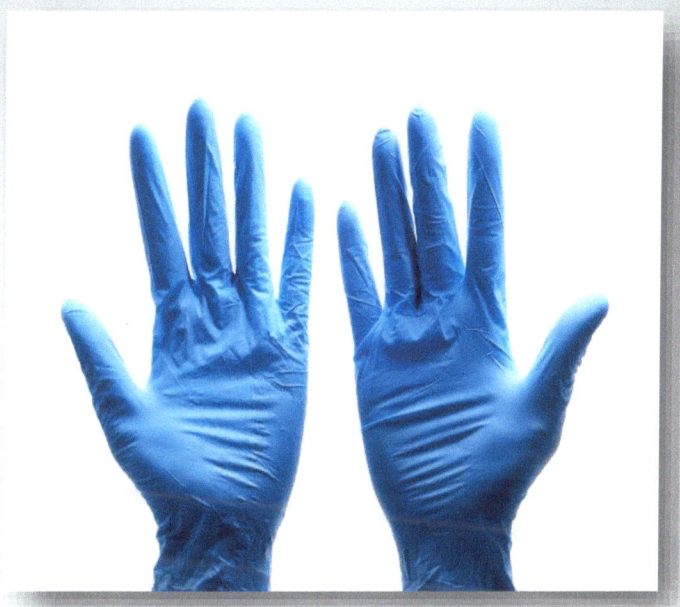

All members of your health care team
Will put on gloves to protect you

Wearing gloves will keep their hands clean
So they will not infect you.

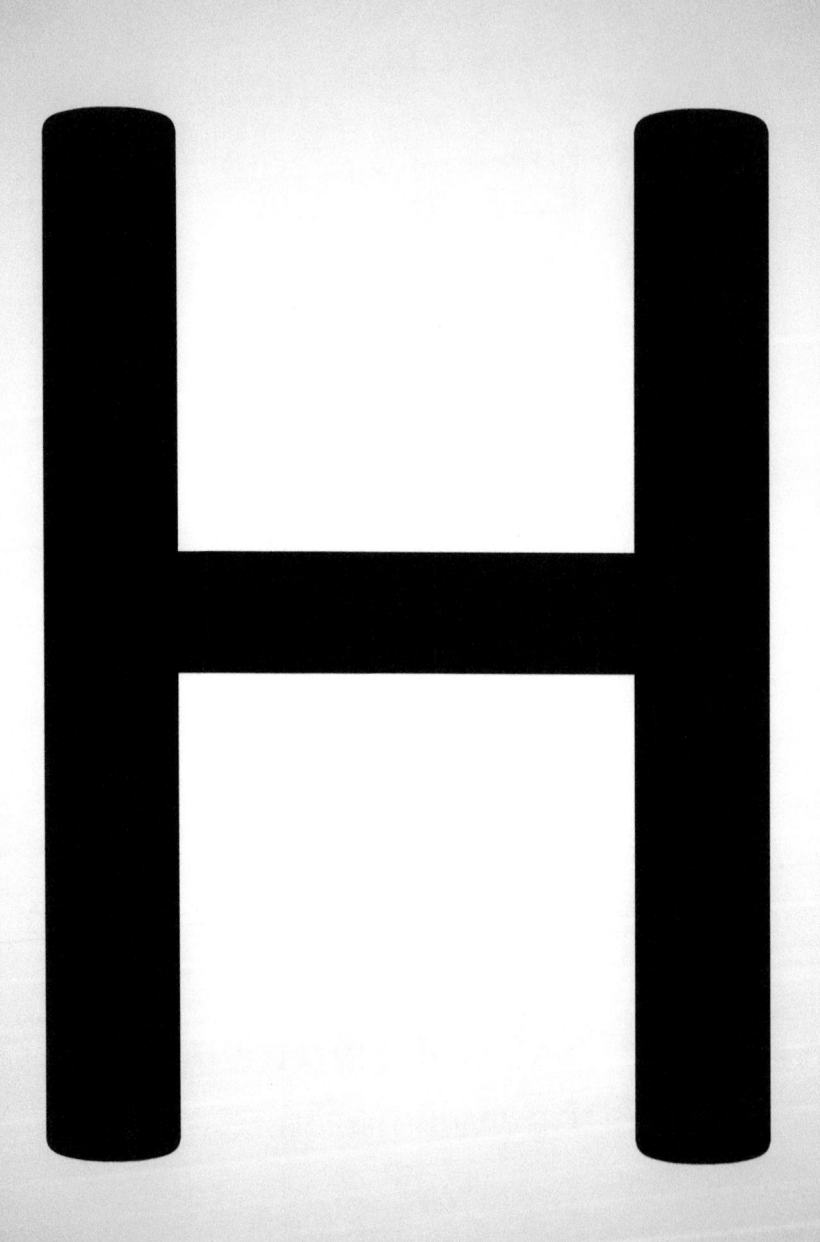

H: Hospital

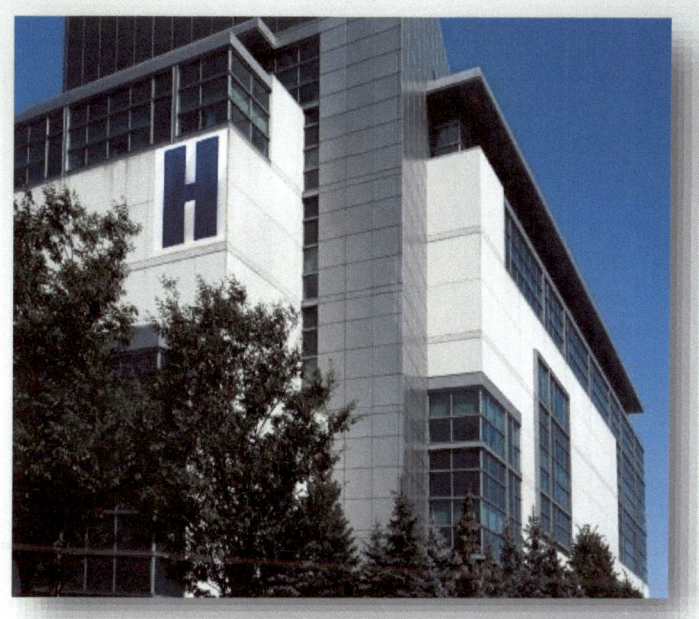

A hospital is a place you may go
To have a special test or visit someone you know

You may have to sleep there so the staff can get you well
Then you can return to home feeling swell!

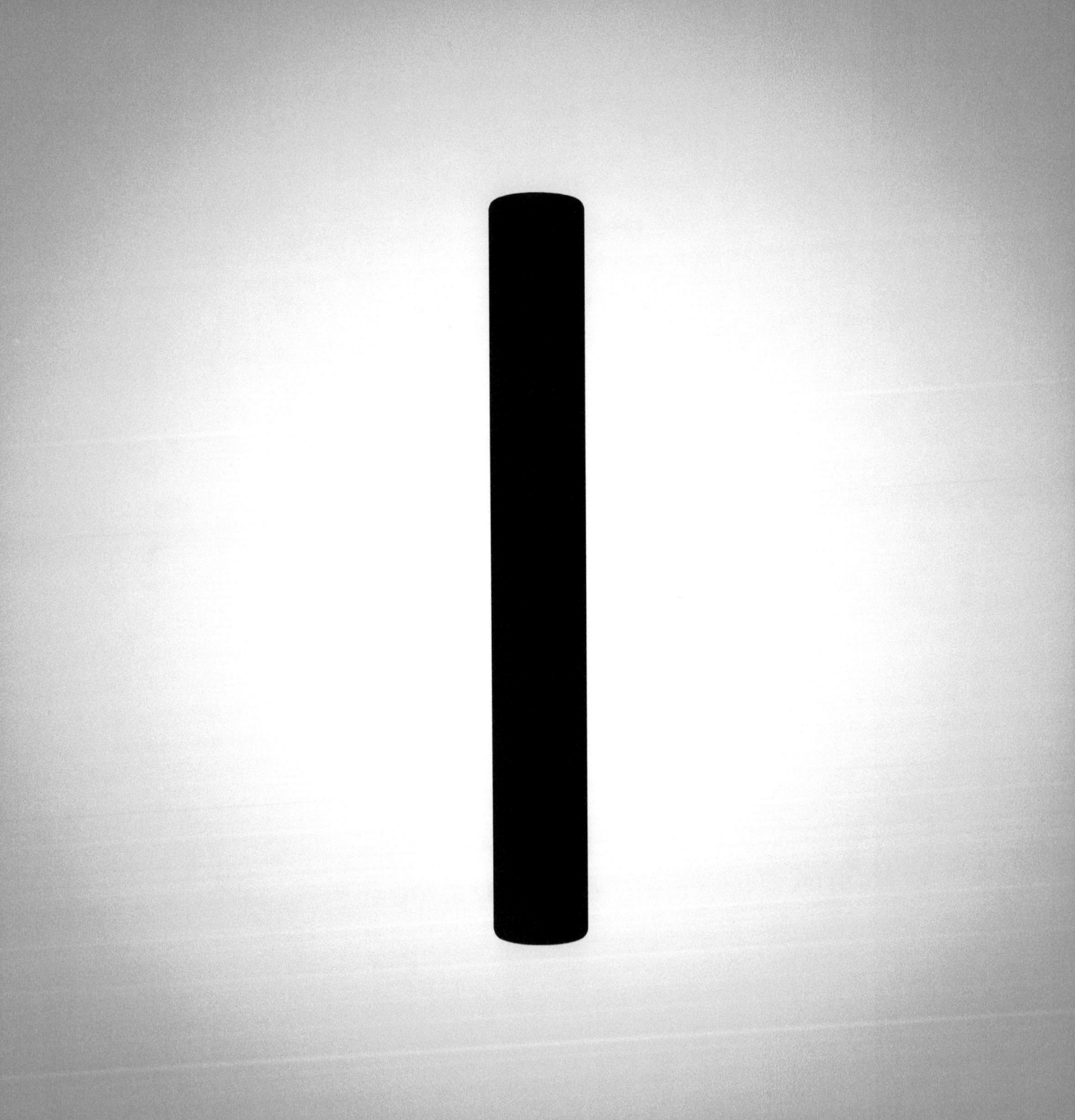

I: Intravenous (IV)

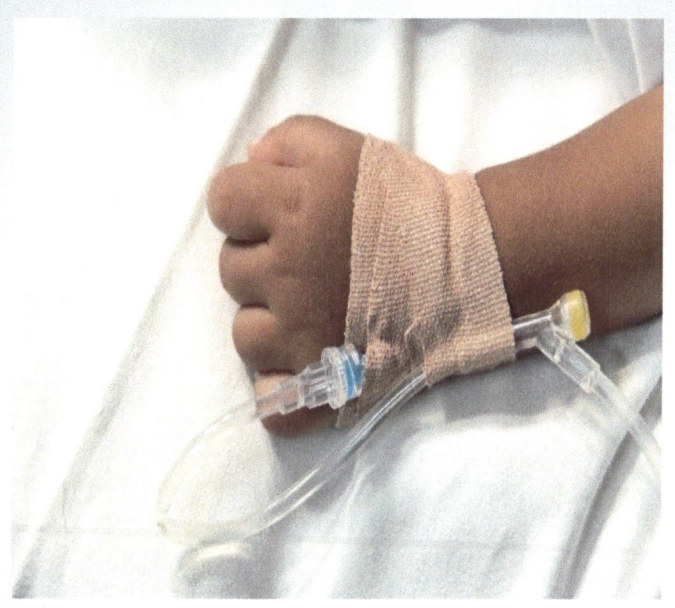

If you need special medicine or if your tank is low
You may need an IV because that is the best way to go

Once it is placed the nurses know
To start the fluid and let it flow.

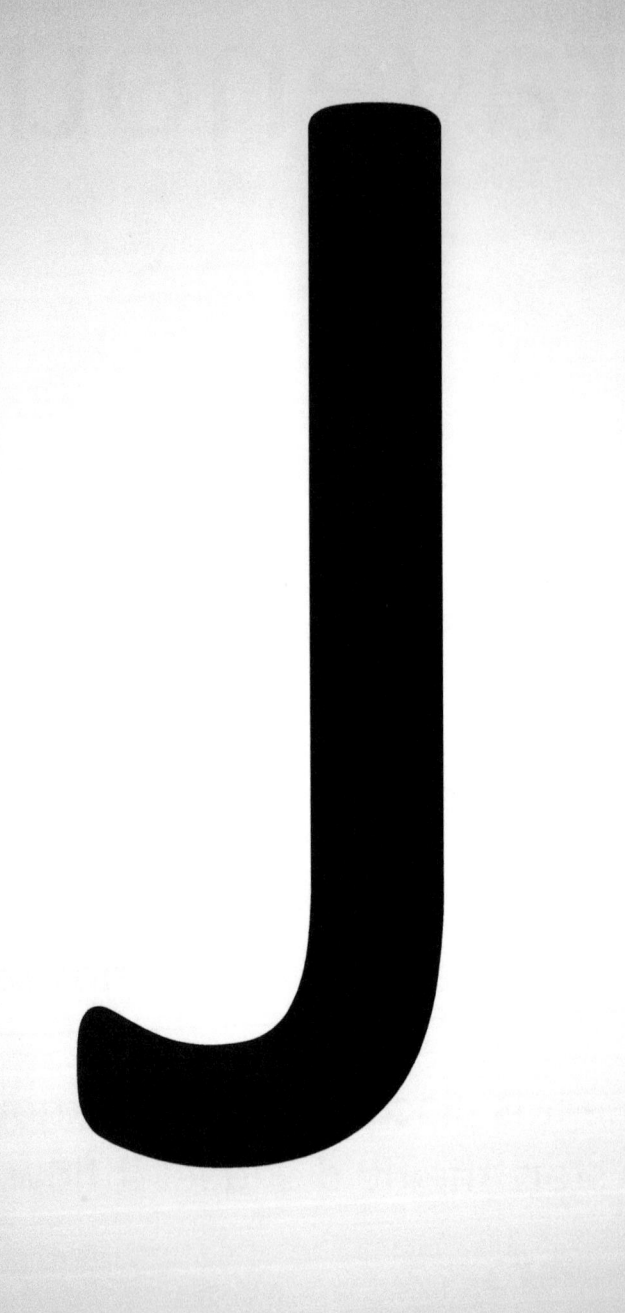

J: Jello

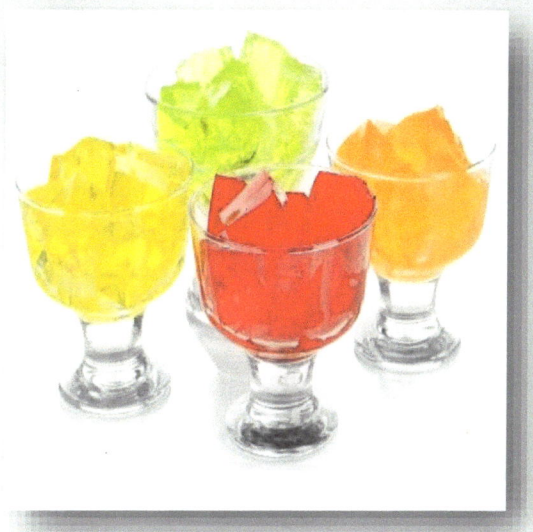

Sometimes when you are not feeling well
You may be given something cold that looks like a gel

It comes in many colors, like red, green and yellow
It is easy to eat and we call it JELLO!

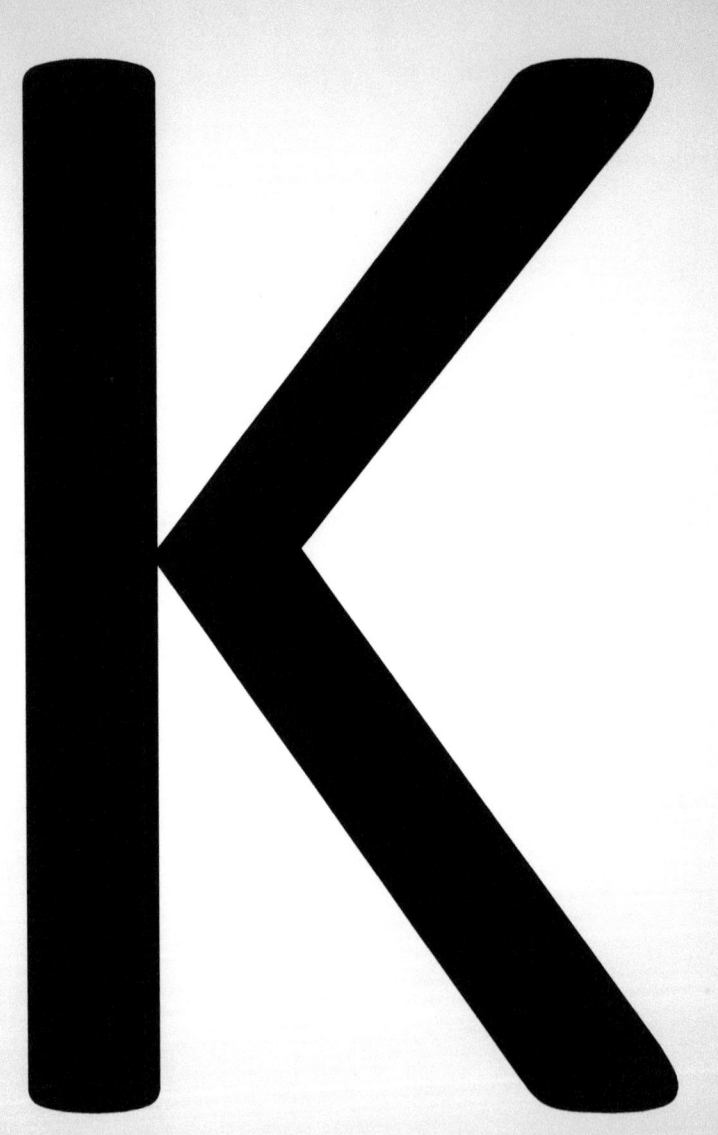

K: Kilogram

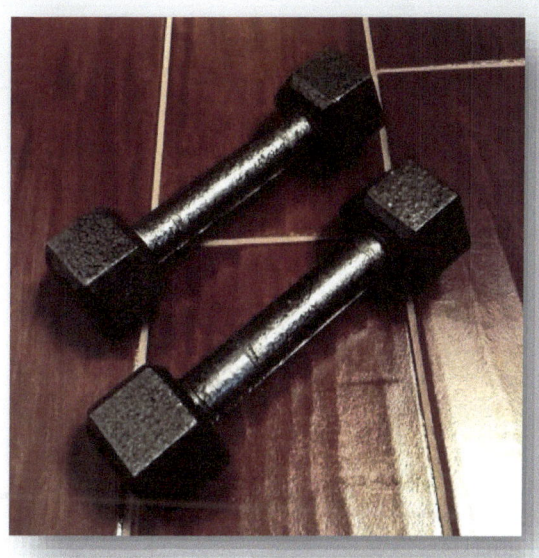

A kilogram is a unit of measure
That is used to chart your weight

One kilogram is equal to 2.2 pounds
It will tell us your growing rate.

1 kilogram = 2.2 pounds

L: Litter

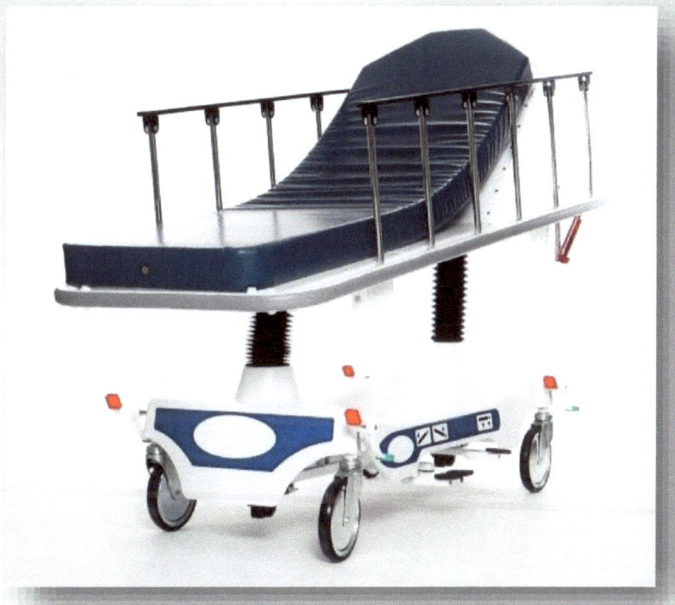

A litter in the hospital is a bed on wheels
You will ride on it to every test

Litters are very comfortable
On it you will be able to rest.

M

M: Mask

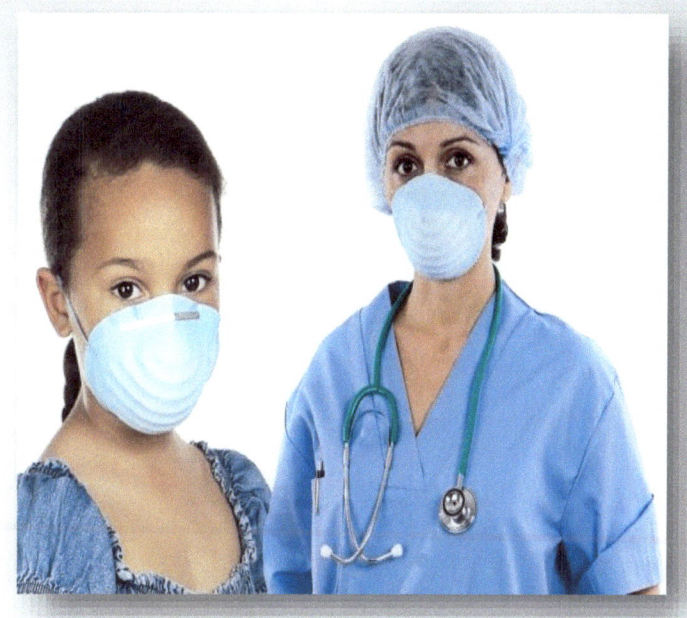

A hospital mask protects you from germs
In the back of the head it ties

The mask will cover most of your face
But you can still see with your eyes.

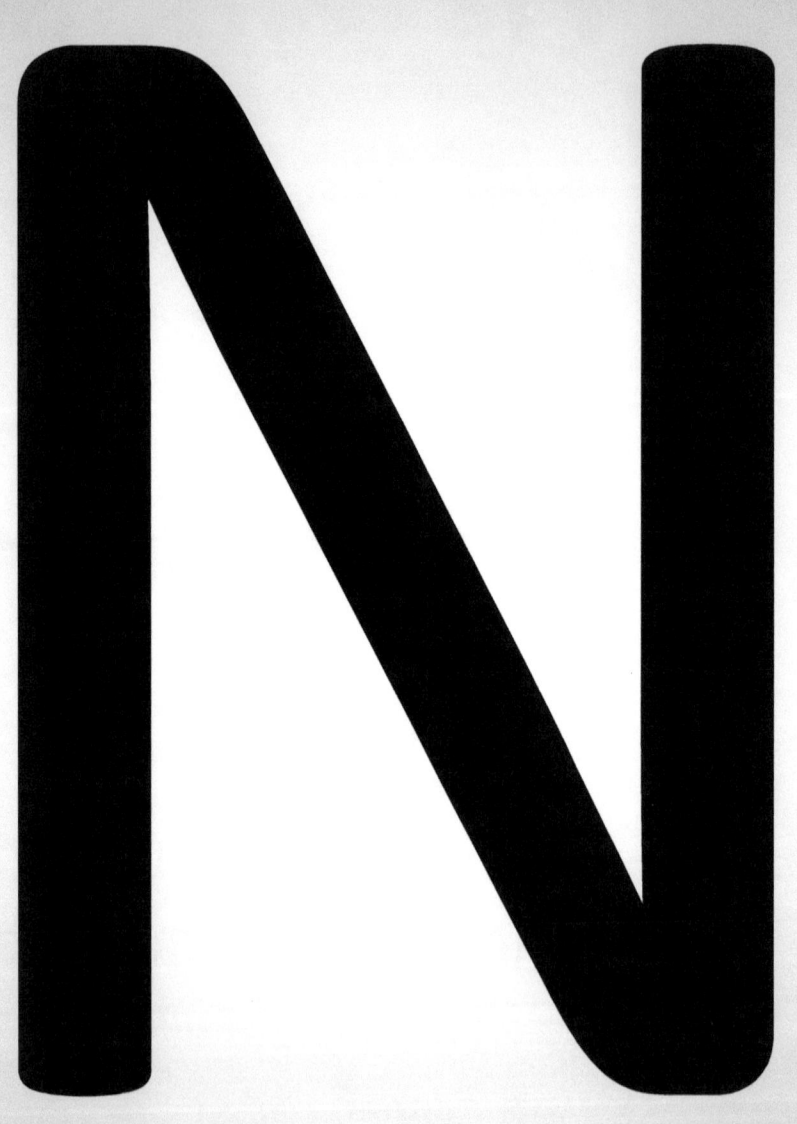

N: Needle

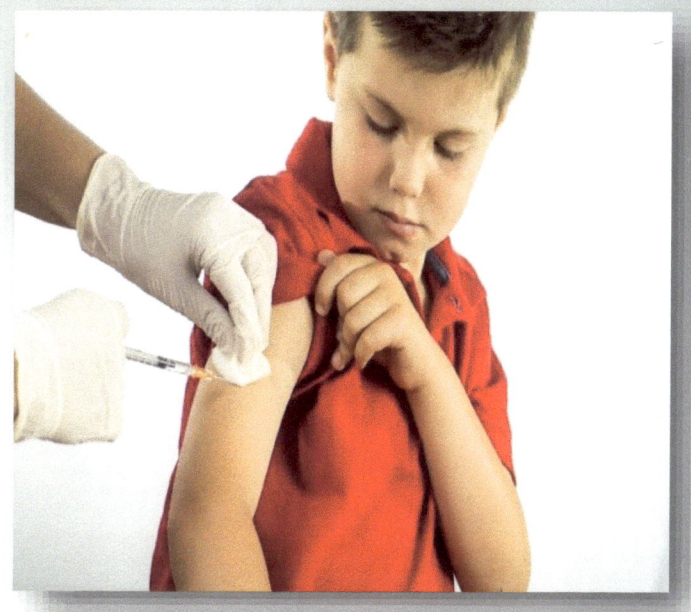

A needle is necessary to give us medicine
Its purpose is to keep us well

It does hurt for a brief moment
But after you can hardly tell.

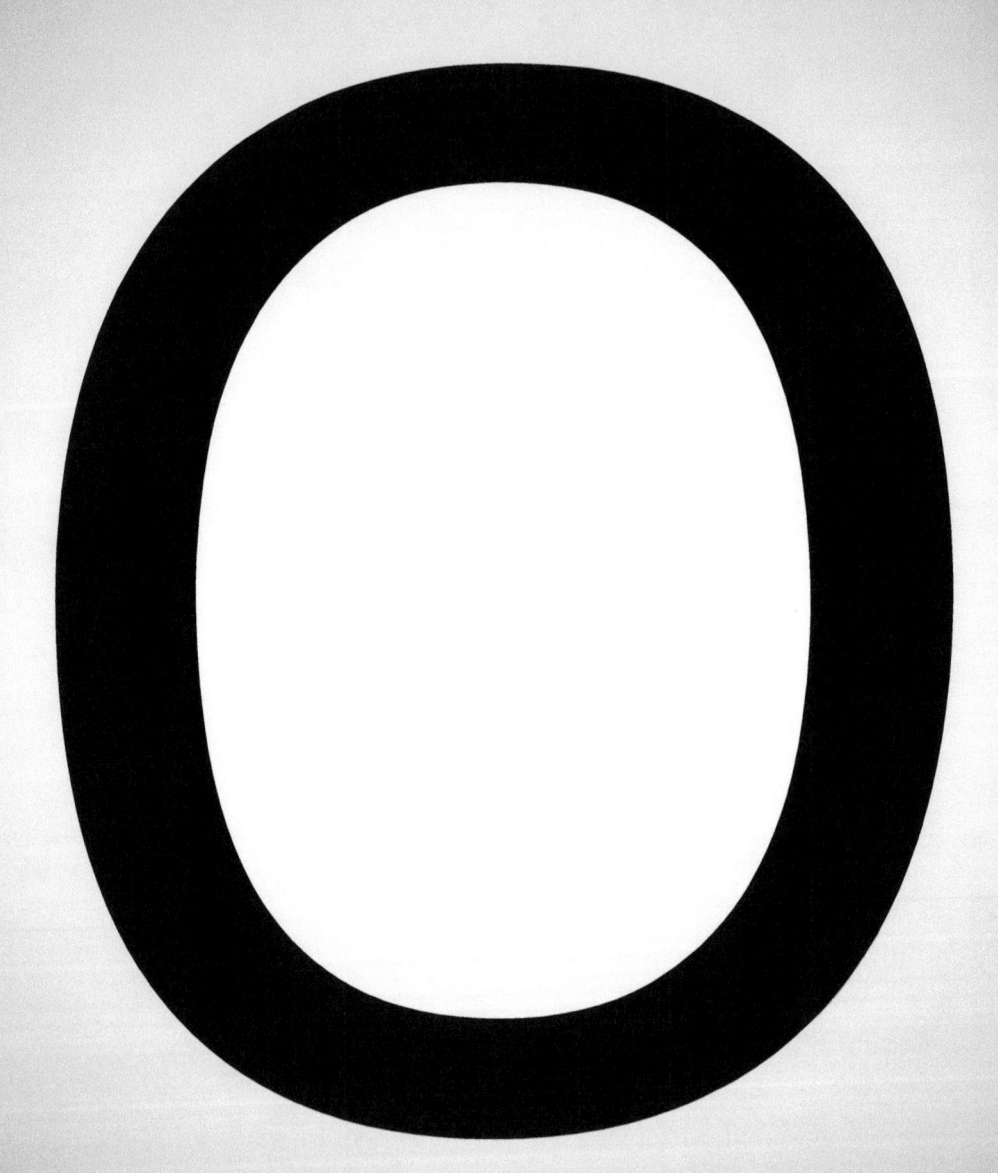

O: Oxygen

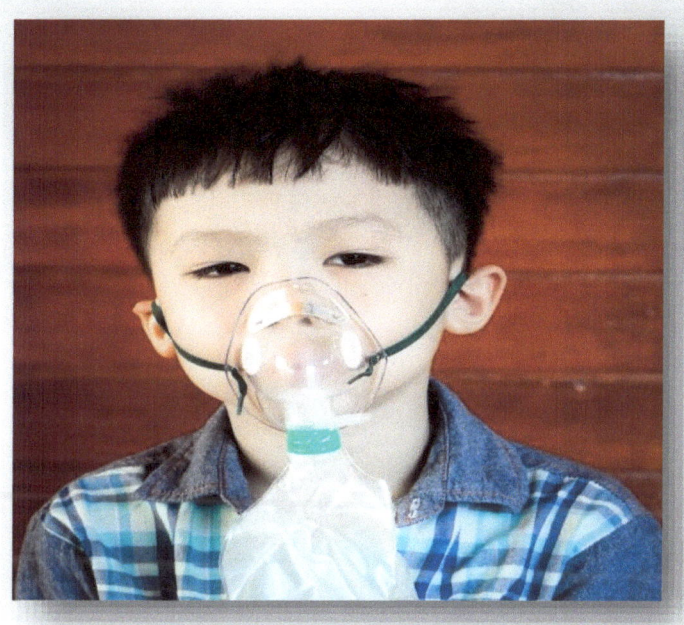

Oxygen is found in the air
We breathe it in without a care

If we have a problem with our lungs
We may need extra given by a mask or nasal prongs.

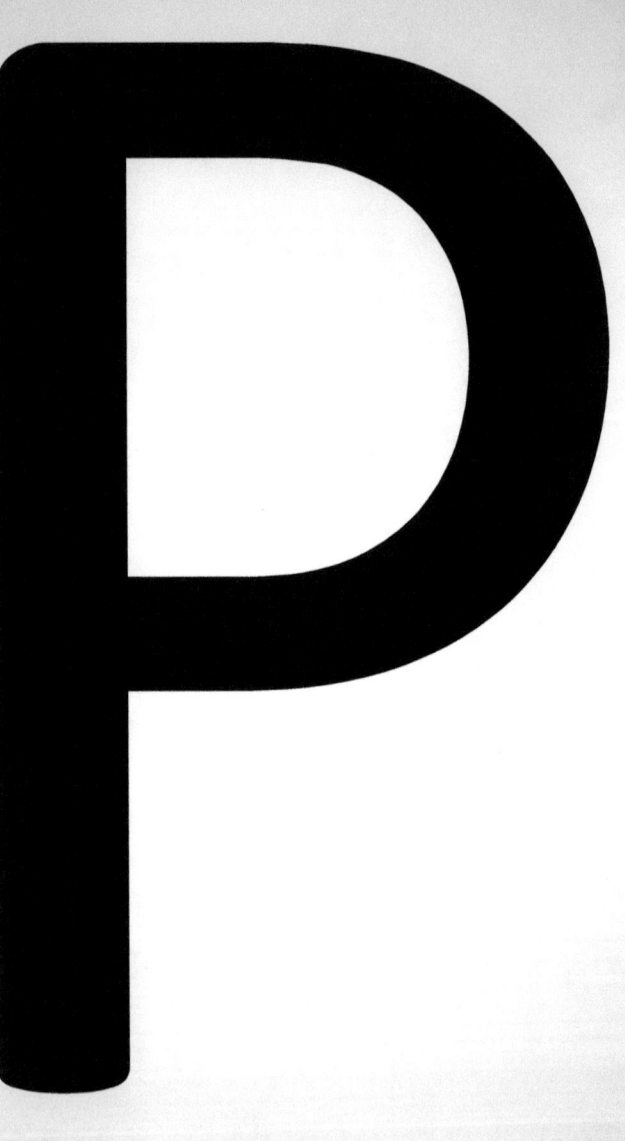

P: Pulse

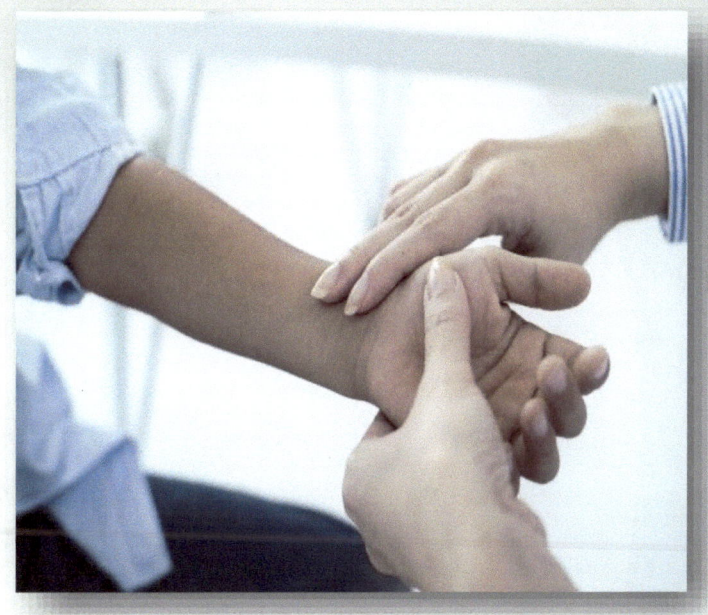

A pulse is also called a heartbeat
We feel in our wrists, neck, or on top of our feet

We count the number of beats per minute
The number is checked to see if it is within our age limit.

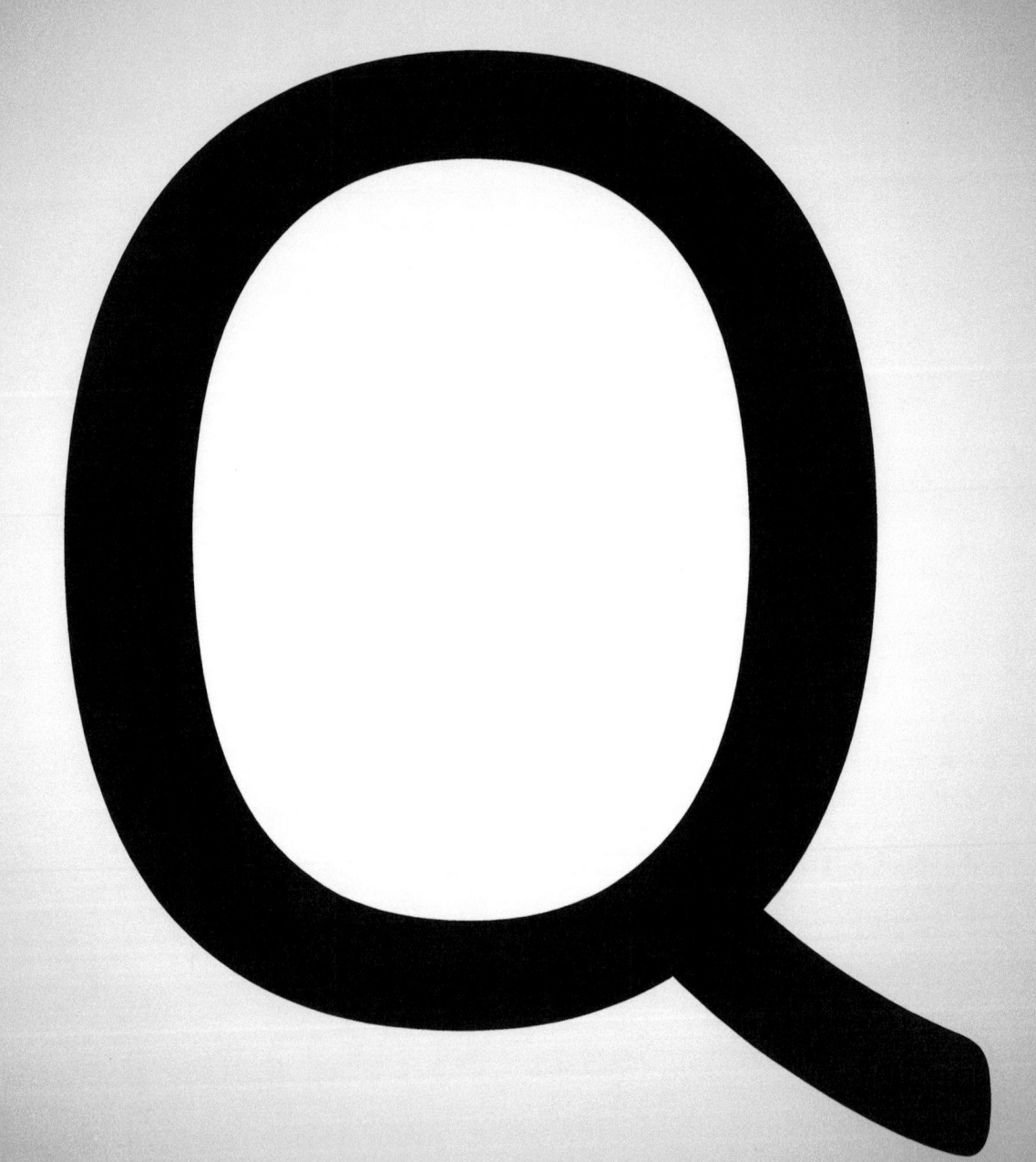

Q: Qtip

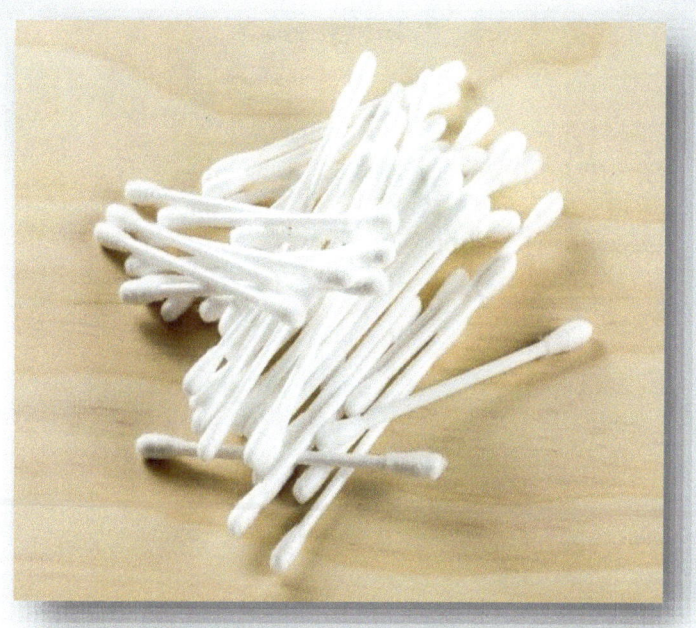

A Qtip can also be called a cotton swab
It is used to clean your outer ear and does a great job

Can be used to apply ointment on an abrasion or tear
It is soft and always used with care.

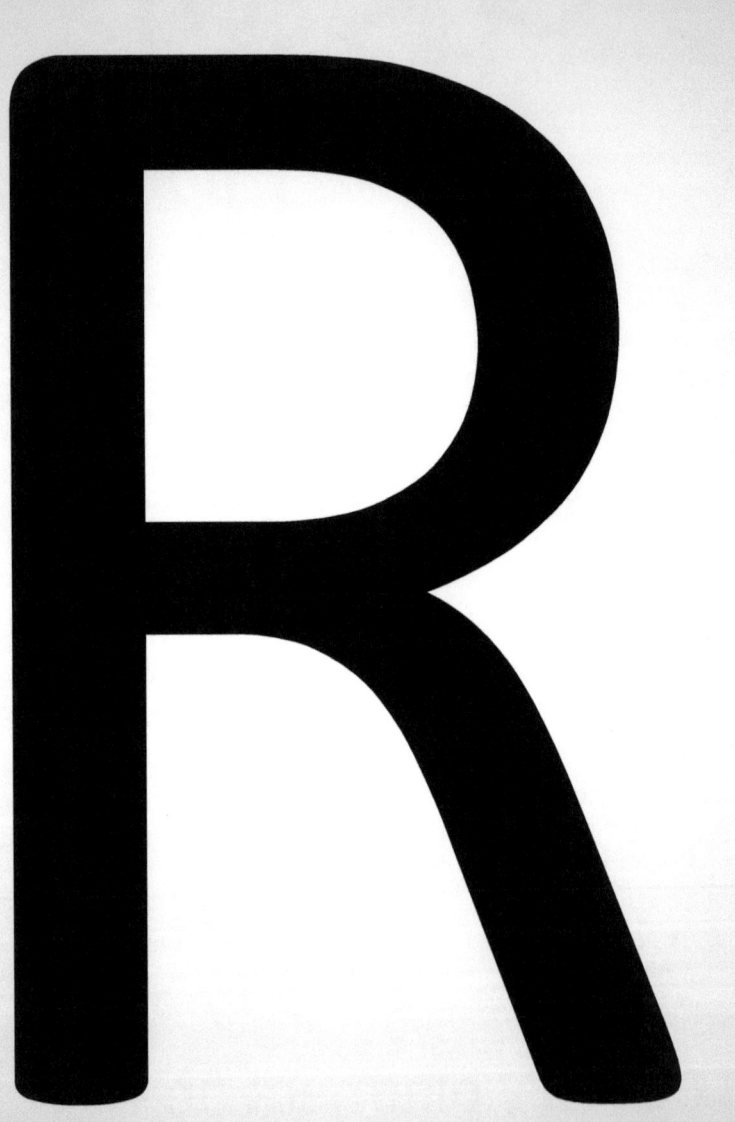

R: Radiology

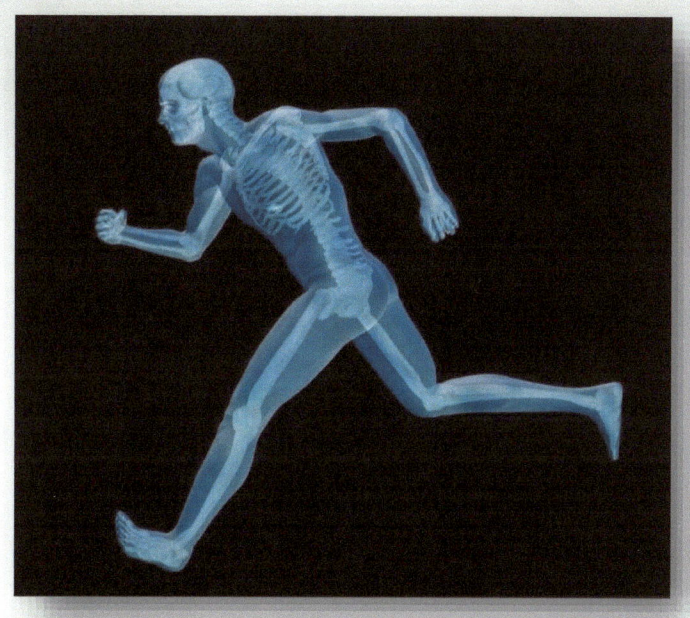

A word you may hear is Radiology
This department is full of technology

Pictures of your body we will take
To view the inside where it may ache.

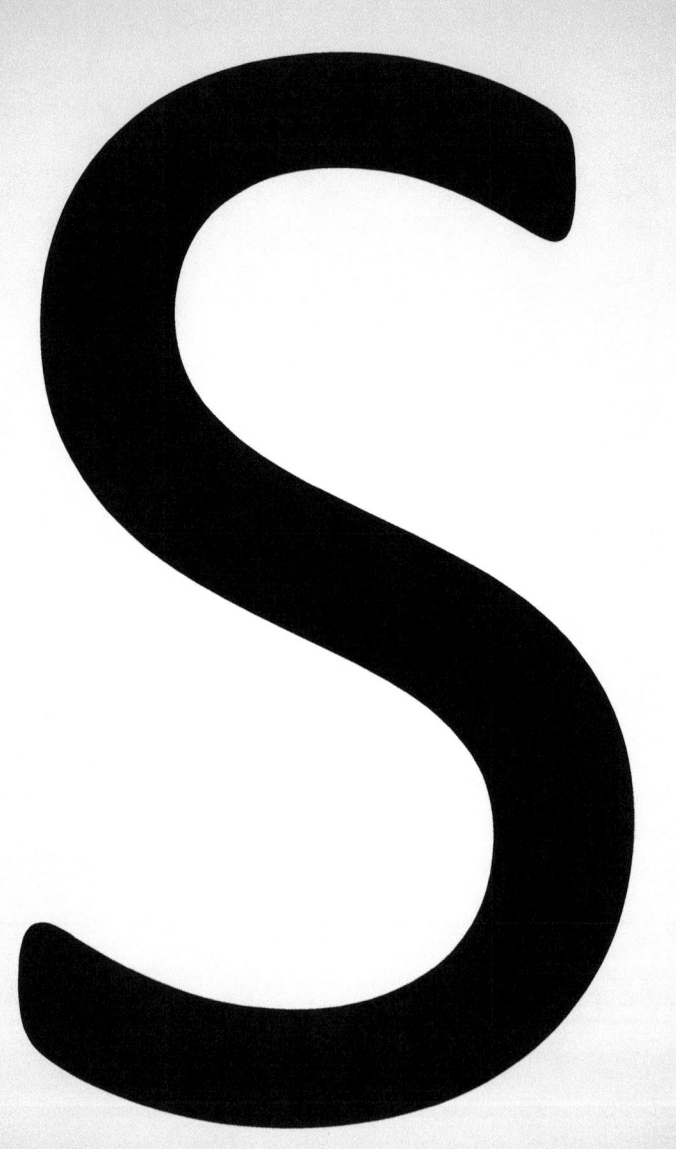

S: Scale

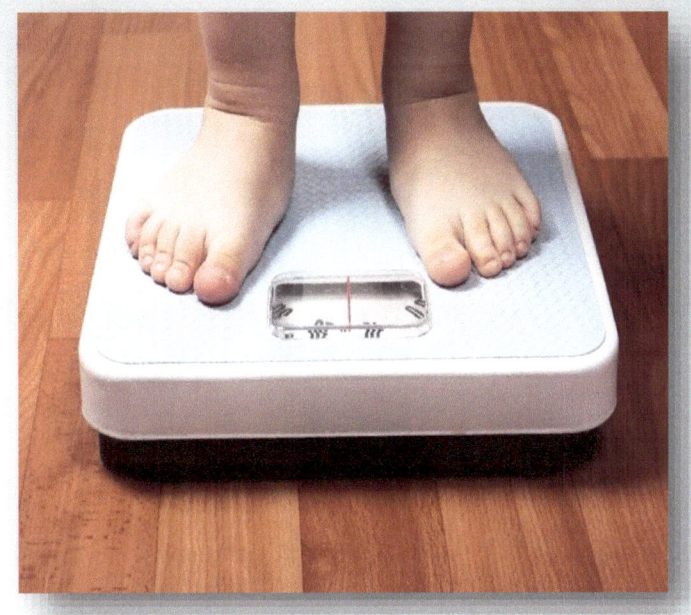

A scale is used to measure your weight
Recorded in kilograms or pounds

Whatever size you are is just right
Because you are growing by leaps and bounds.

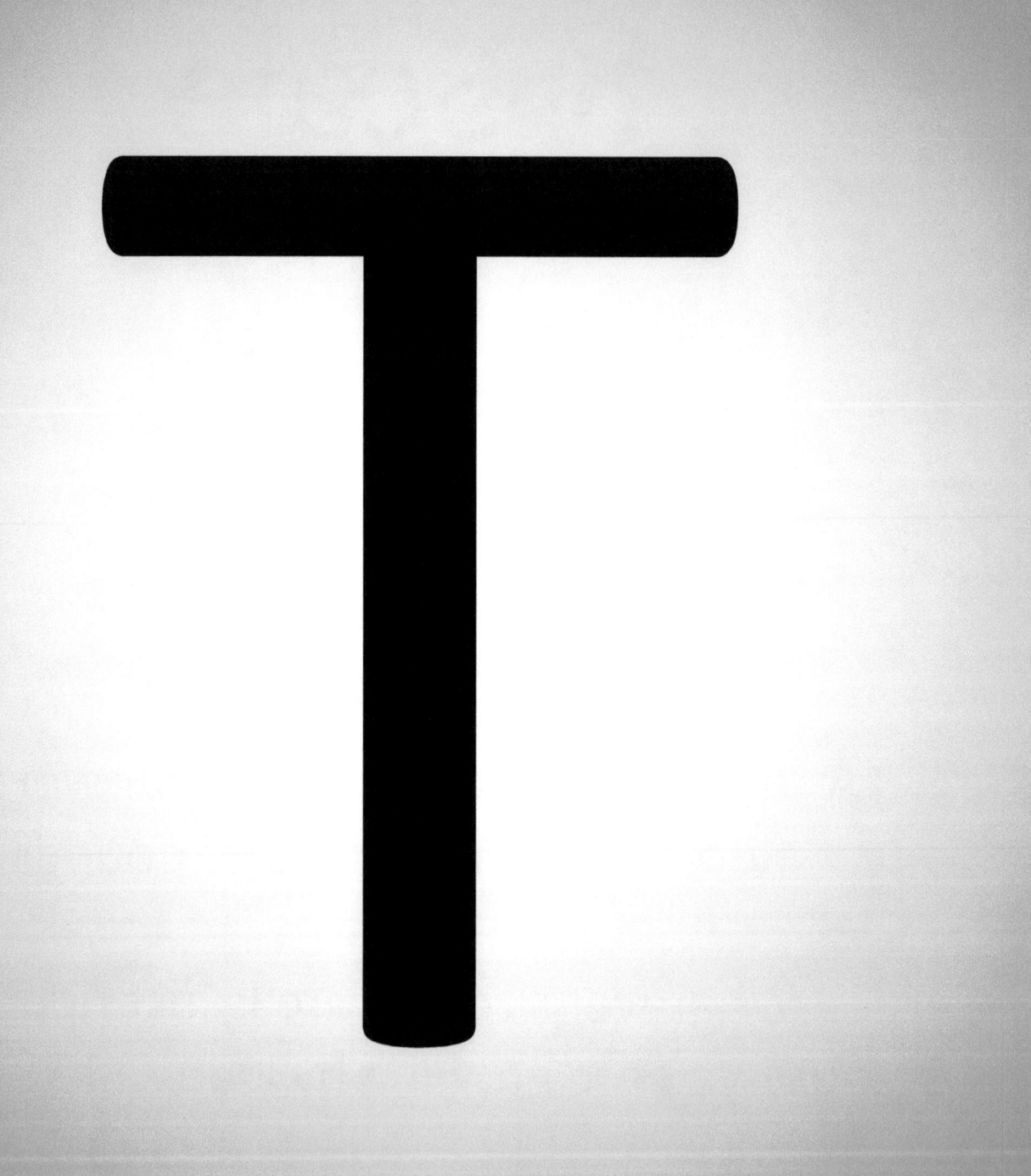

T: Thermometer

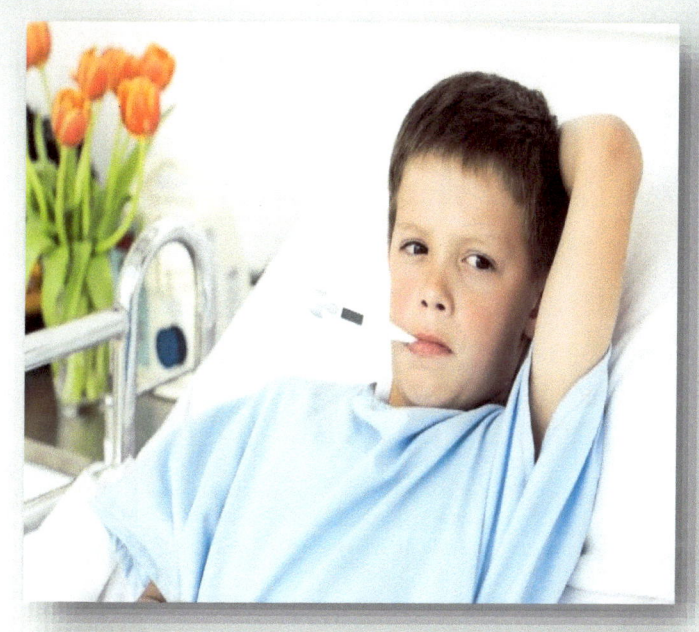

Your temperature is measured with a thermometer
In degrees called Celsius or Fahrenheit

We place it in your ear or under your tongue
So we make sure we get the numbers right.

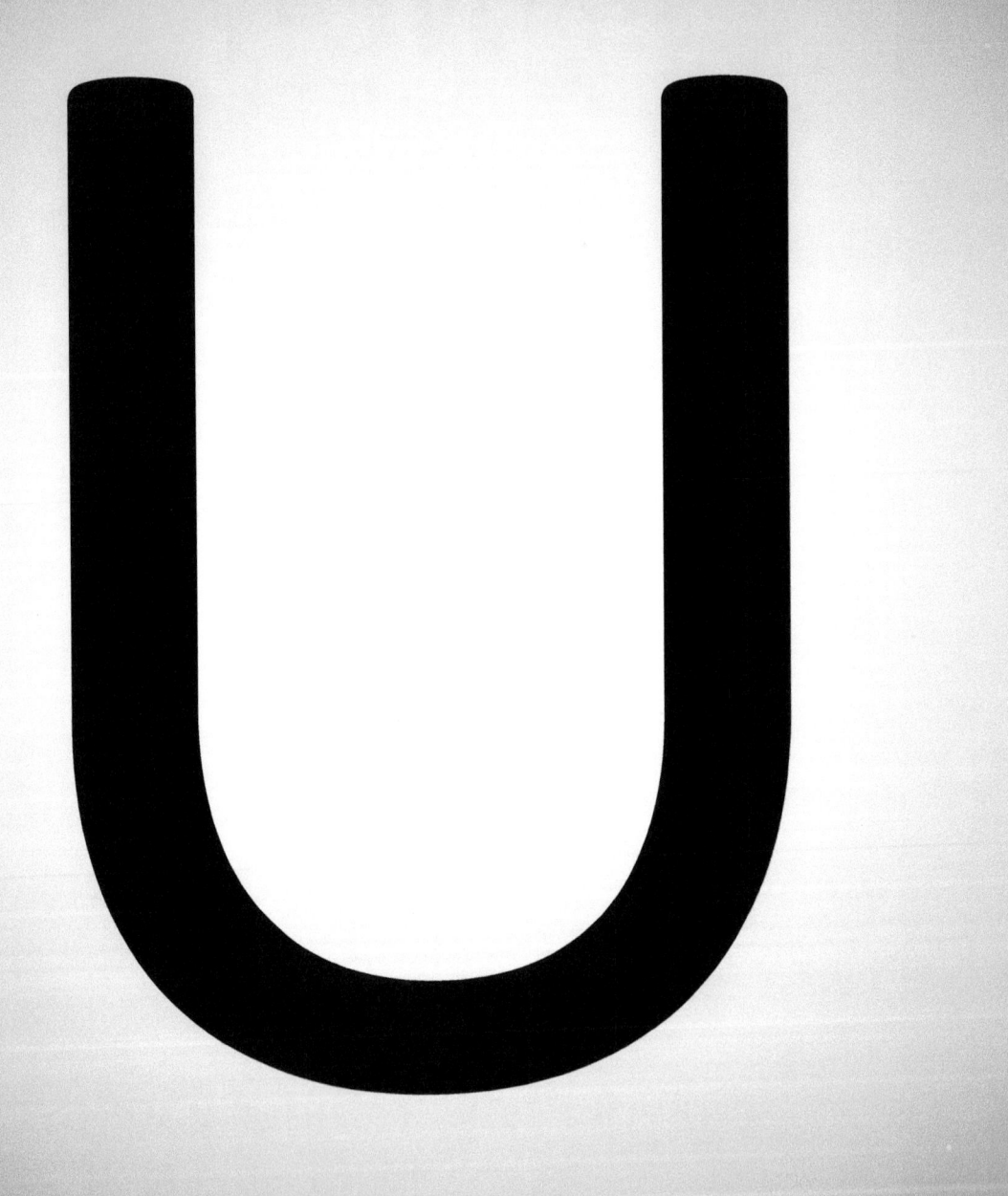

U: Urgent Care

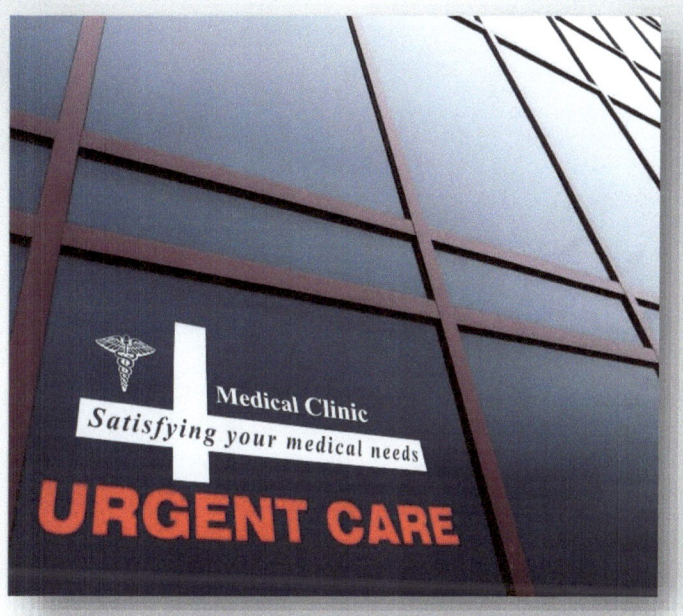

Urgent Care is a place you go
If you need help really quick

There are professional medical people there
That can help you when you are injured or sick.

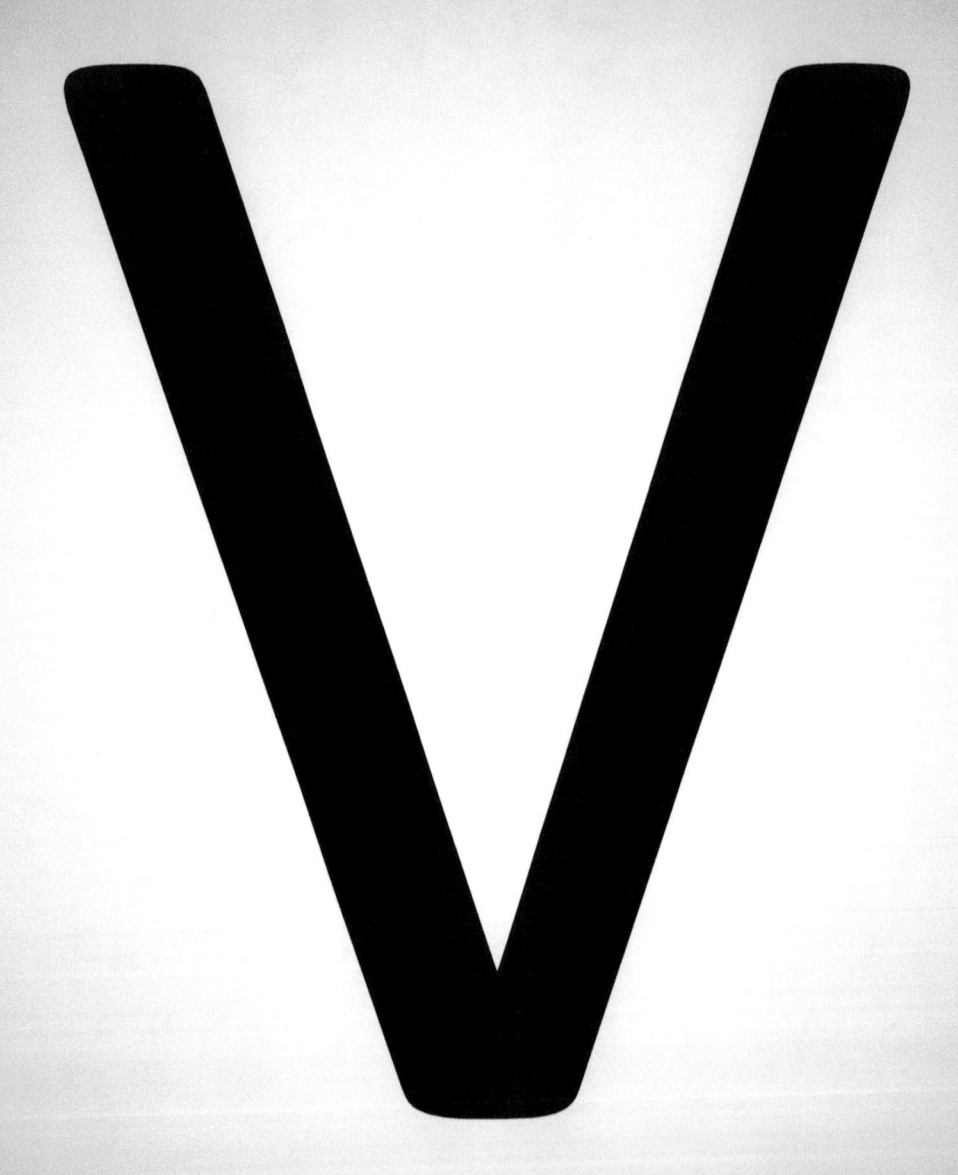

V: Vision Chart

A Vision Chart is used to check your eyes
It tests the sharpness of your vision

The chart contains letters of all different sizes
The goal is to evaluate your visual precision.

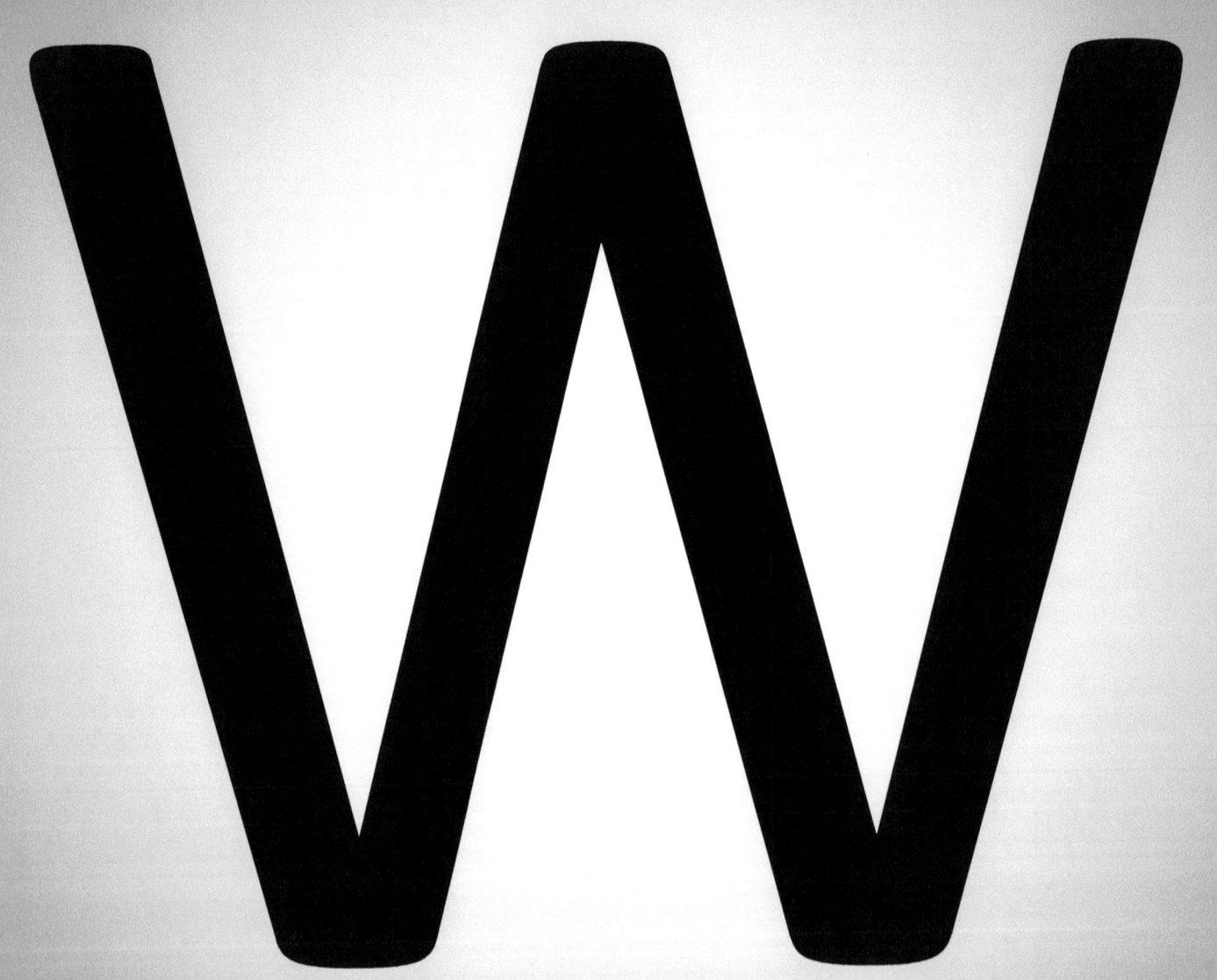

W: Wheelchair

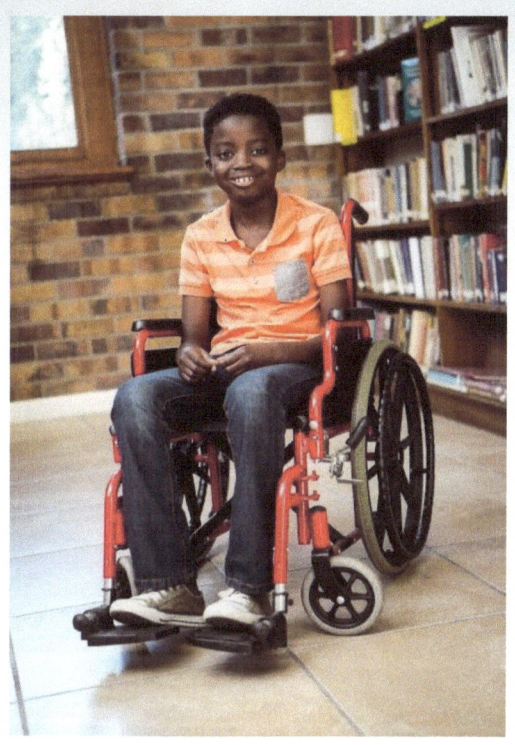

If your legs are hurt or your body is weak
You may have to take a special seat

There is a chair with wheels below
It will transport where you need to go.

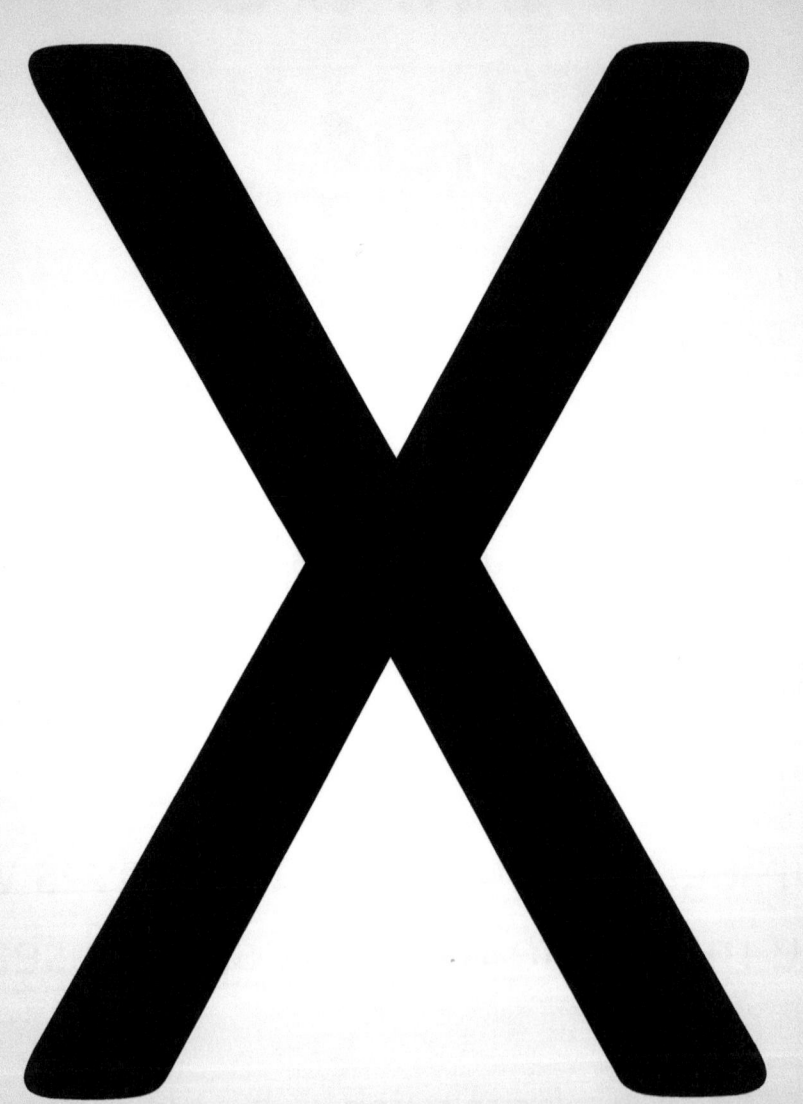

X: Xray

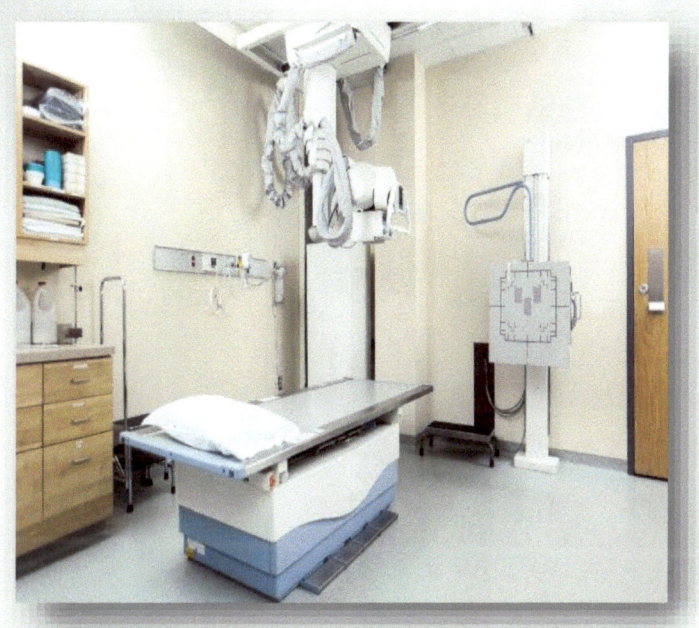

An Xray will need to be taken
If you have a body part that may be aching

Inside of your body we will be able to see
This helps us to know what the problem maybe.

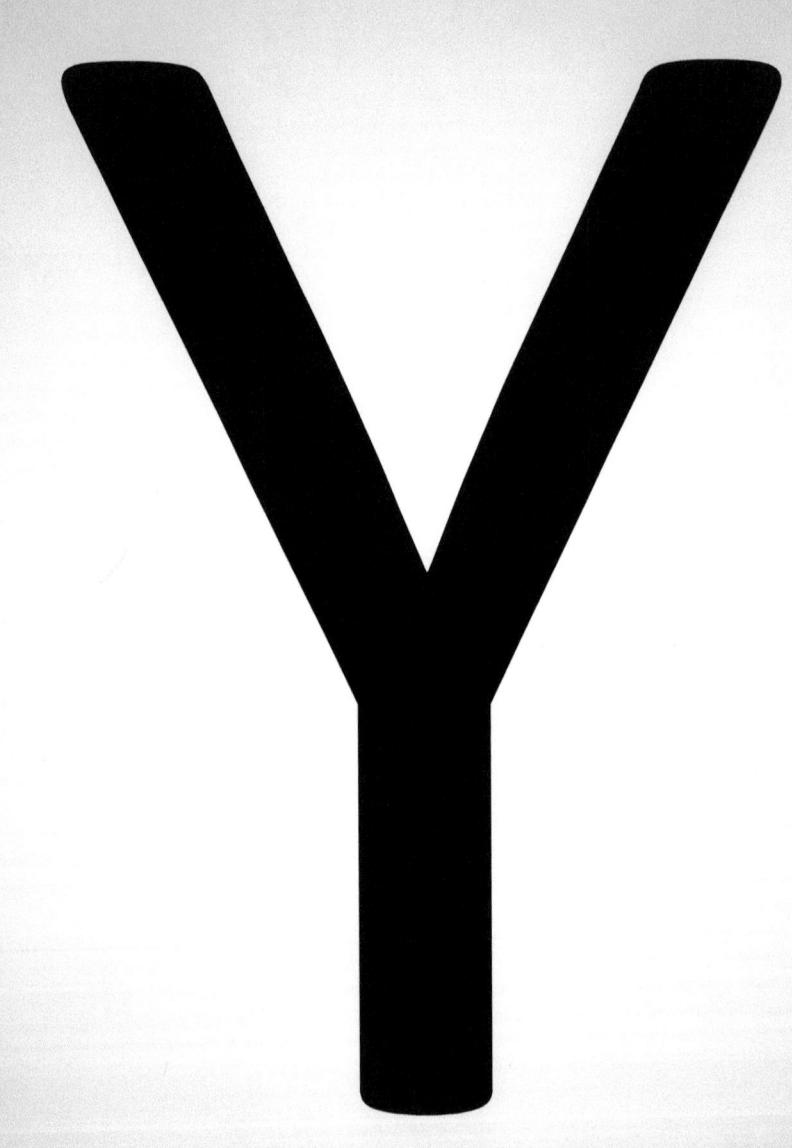

Y: Yankauer (yang- kow-er)

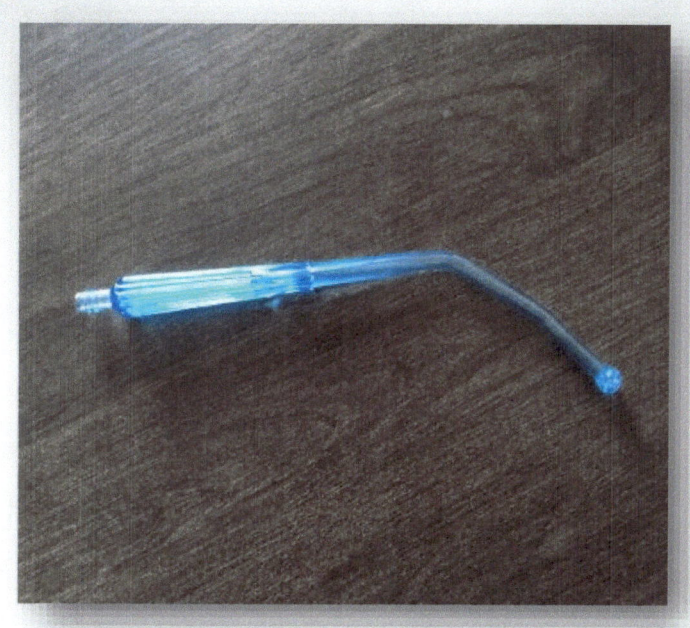

A Yankauer has suction that goes in your mouth
It helps to get the oral secretions out

This tool removes your saliva or spit
Used in the hospital or dentist office when you need it.

Z:

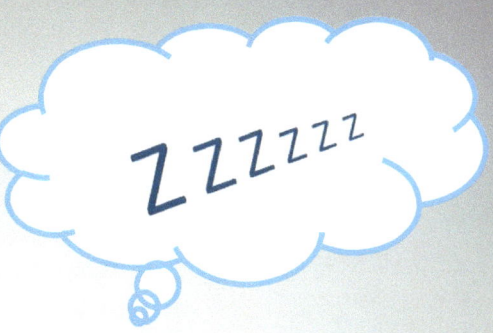

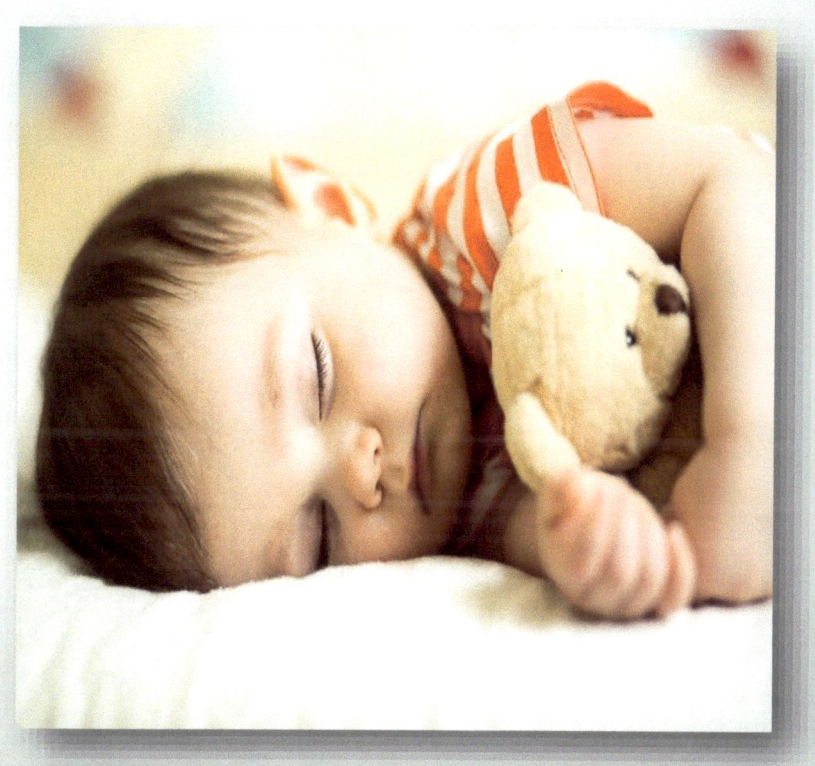

Goodnight!

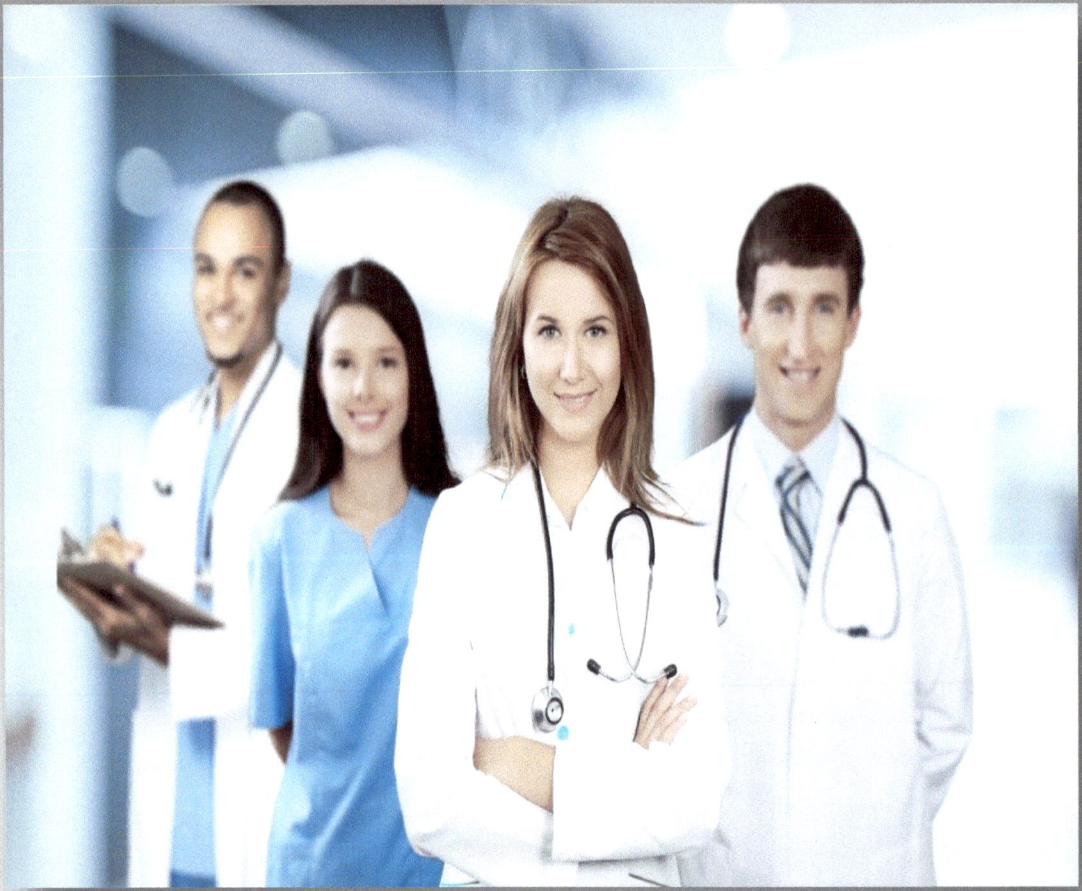

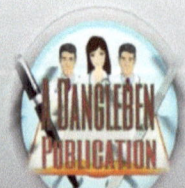

You also will see
a whole bunch of smiling faces
wherever you will be!